The Bridal diet

Also by the same author
Lose a Kilo a Week

The *Bridal* diet

Nishi Grover

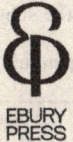

EBURY
PRESS

An imprint of Penguin Random House

EBURY PRESS

USA | Canada | UK | Ireland | Australia
New Zealand | India | South Africa | China | Singapore

Ebury Press is part of the Penguin Random House group of companies
whose addresses can be found at global.penguinrandomhouse.com

Published by Penguin Random House India Pvt. Ltd
4th Floor, Capital Tower 1, MG Road,
Gurugram 122 002, Haryana, India

Penguin
Random House
India

First published by Random House India 2015

10 9 8 7 6 5 4 3

ISBN 9788184006629

Photography: Tara Upadhyay
Model: Tarini Uppal

Typeset in Requiem Text by Manipal Digital Systems, Manipal

Printed at Repro India Limited

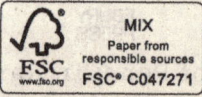
This is a legitimate digitally printed version of the book and therefore might not
have certain extra finishing on the cover.

To my father Dr Ashok Grover, my mother Mrs Uma Grover, my sister Neelima Grover, and my brother Dr Varun Grover, for all their love and support

Contents

Contents

Introduction

'Every bride is beautiful. It's like newborn babies or puppies.
They can't help it'—**Emme Rollins**, *Dear Rockstar*

Did you read the quote above?

Isn't it so true? Every bride *is* beautiful. Why won't she be? After all, her wedding day is one of the most important events of her life. It marks the day when she transforms into a woman. And that itself is enough to make her glow. But why then am I writing this book?

After the success of *Lose a Kilo a Week,* I was flooded with calls and emails from people wanting more. And I noticed that a lot of the calls were from brides-to-be, calling in to get me to get them in fabulous shape before their wedding. A few even called me two weeks before the big day! Now, I was able to help them out as much as I could but I'm not a magician who can transform you into Cinderella's alter ego if you give me a second to do it!

This got me thinking about the pressures of the wedding day. In Delhi itself, come the winter months, I attend countless weddings each year. And every year I hear the same story from brides and grooms who want to be fit before the main day. As weddings become more Bollywood inspired and grow more and more glamorous each year, the pressure on the brides to look smashing and put up the best show in town has become enormously high.

Gone are the days when a wedding was managed by just the members of your family. Now it's all destination weddings, and theme weddings, and whatnot. Spas and salons today even have packages exclusively tailored for brides. Before the wedding, brides get into a frenzy, a helter-skelter panic of juicing, heavy gym sessions, crash diets and visits to the parlour. But in all of this we're missing a vital link. If you were keeping fit and eating the right foods all year round, you would never have to resort to the mad rush of activities that befall all brides. This simple truth is often forgotten in our daily lives. So in this book, I want to outline a beauty programme aimed at women so that the days leading up to their wedding can be fun and spared for other activities, such as shopping! ☺

If you have read *Lose a Kilo a Week,* then you will know my background and history, and why I got into fitness and nutrition. My journey has been a long and arduous one, filled with visits to the hospital. At the age of four, I was diagnosed with Type 1 diabetes along with a host of other complications. While other children scampered about and ate candies and cake, I had to come to terms with the fact that my body was different—vulnerable and brittle. I embraced the concept of being nutritionally sound and physically fit and made it a part of my life. This was my battle and I had every intention of fighting it tooth and nail. Over the years, I learnt something from every client who walked in through the door at my clinic. They all had a story of how they perceived food, and why they ate. It was a long educating process for me. However, I saw a pattern in my clients, and I understood what led people to eat the way they did. Today, my 1000-plus clients swear by me. They keep coming back, bringing friends, relatives, spouses along with them to join my programme. And they do it for a reason—my programme works. It is simple, logical and successful. Most importantly, it hasn't ever changed because the needs of the human body will never change. The basic physiological and chemical make-up of a body requires a few fundamental elements to let it function smoothly, including the right kind of food. For example, you need 70 per cent of carbohydrates, 20 per cent of protein, and the remaining 10 per cent of sugars, fats, minerals and vitamins in your diet. If you give your body the above you have done 80 per cent of the job of living healthy. The remaining 20 per cent is a good lifestyle and exercise.

A Book for Everyone

Even though this book focuses on the wedding belles, it really is for everyone. Because health is not just for those who are about to get married. Even if you aren't getting hitched, you can still use this book to get in shape and get fit. Because a fit body is an investment everyone should make. So go ahead, and give it a try. In this book, I show you how to eat right and live right. People often forget that sometimes the answers lie in the simplest things. That the food you're eating can make you fat and can also make you lose weight and bring happiness and well-being in your life. But more often than not, people lose sight of the details that make up the larger picture. So it's my duty to make them see the light. And once I've done that, it makes me happy to see a transformed happy and healthy person.

In this book, I use my concept of the CCQ diet (low-calorie, low-carbs, low-quantity) combined with exercise to make you a fit and healthy bride. My programme highlights the essential foods you should be eating, when and how much. It also tells you what you're doing wrong, what to avoid and to learn self-control.

If you follow the principles of this book carefully and sincerely I can guarantee that on D-Day you'll be the glowing bride that you seek to be. By reading this book, you've taken the first step to getting there. And I want to congratulate you for taking this road to a healthy life (and on your wedding!). The first step may seem daunting, but persist and you will see results. Everything comes to the one who is true and sincere. The words may seem false in our modern world, but don't let its simplicity fool you.

This book celebrates a new beginning, one in which you will shine like stars in the night sky. As every happy and healthy bride deserves.

How to Use this Book

I have divided the book into four parts. Each part deals with a particular practical topic. This is designed so that the book is easy to use and reference is easy after you're done reading.

Part I explains the dietary problems particular to girls who are about to get married. World-over weddings have become high-pressure events, where the focus is more on looking good and keeping up with the Joneses rather than the actual ceremony itself. The pressures of looking their best on D-Day takes today's girls on dangerous crash diets and juicing programmes, which ultimately cause more harm than good. In this part I also explain the philosophy behind the beautiful bride programme, which is the foundation of my teachings. Once that is clear, I suggest you move onto the next part. Here's a breakdown of what each chapter discusses:

In **Chapter 1: Heavier Ever After and Other Troubles** I talk about the Indian wedding scene, the pressure that brides face, and the perils involved in crash dieting.

Chapter 2: Are you Bridelicious? This chapter has a short quiz that evaluates and assesses where you stand health-wise, and what you should be aiming for.

Chapter 3: The Beautiful Bride Programme This chapter is the core of this book. It outlines my health philosophy, how to lose weight, and the how and when to eat. If you grasp this and make it a part of your lifestyle, there'll be no turning back from here on.

Chapter 4: 'I Do . . . Not'—Learning to Say No This is a crucial chapter because most of us cannot say no to food and food pushers. Here I discuss and teach you how to avoid temptation and say no effortlessly.

Part II discusses the foods that we will be eating in the diet and the foods that need to be eliminated. It is a hands-on practical section that is tailored to your needs, and discusses the number of calories you need to burn or the number of kilos you need to shed before your big day. Packed with diet charts and a treasure trove of oil-free recipes, this is the core of the book which will determine your diet programme.

In **Chapter 5: The Wedding Planner—Getting Started** I discuss how to plan getting in shape for your wedding. It involves setting goals, motivation tips and working backwards.

Chapter 6: Diet Plan #1—Losing up to 5 kilos This chapter is tailored for those of you who need to lose up to 5 kilos. The diet charts indicate what your food intake should be like and what kind of foods you should be eating during the given time period.

Chapter 7: Diet Plan #2—Losing Between 5 to 10 kilos This chapter is aimed specifically at those of you who want to lose weight up to 10 kilos, and include diet charts for a given duration.

Chapter 8: Diet Plan #3—Losing Between 10 to 20 kilos Here's another chapter that includes tailored diet plans for those of you who want to lose weight up to 20 kilos.

Chapter 9: Oil-free Recipes for a Beautiful Bride I've included a whole chapter of delicious oil-free recipes to help you on your journey to a healthy and happy you.

Part III tackles the problem areas of most women—arms, legs, the bum and the tummy—with easy and effective exercises that can be done in the comfort of your own home. This is a crucial section of the book, as no diet is ever truly effective without a workout programme. The workouts are short and basic, but combined with the diet they will give you the maximum results.

Chapter 10: Getting Workout Ready This chapter takes you through the prep work required to start your fitness programme. Remember, your diet plan falls flat without a workout routine to boost it.

Chapter 11: Up in Arms Tackling one of the most common problems faced by women, this chapter shows you the exercises you can do to get toned arms.

Chapter 12: Belle and the Belly In this chapter, we combat the tummy with exercises that will help you show off a flat abdomen in no time.

Chapter 13: The Bottom Line Here I outline an exercise routine that will firm your behind and help you get into those skinny jeans without much wriggling.

Chapter 14: Shake a Leg Another problem area, another chapter! Once again, I've outlined a workout routine to get your legs firm and toned in time for the big day.

Part IV is the maintenance part of the book. Here I talk about one of the most important problems faced by women—putting on weight after marriage. This is such a common problem that a sizable chunk of my clients come to me with this. I discuss ways to keep off weight, how to not fall into the post-wedding weight-gain trap and how to maintain your general good health.

Chapter 13: The Honey after the Moon This chapter discusses the weight problems that surface after the wedding and what you can do to check it and be fit.

PART 1

The Philosophy

1

Heavier Ever After and
Other Troubles

> Carrie: 'So really, we're, we're getting married?'
> Mr Big: 'We're getting married. Should we get you a diamond?'
> Carrie: 'No. No. Just get me a really big closet.'
> —**Sex and the City**

The Sixth Season

Here in Delhi, we must talk about the weather first—
since we live under its iron rule. The seasons swing from
one extreme to the other like a pendulum gone mad. The
details of our lives change thoda thoda se every month.
Refreshing nimbu paanis and lassis in May, hearty soups
in January. This also means that we, Dilliwallahs, have
a wardrobe extensive enough to clothe a small country.
Like Bhutan perhaps. But as the cruel summer months
simmer down and the brief monsoon skitters past,
something changes. The weather mellows, tempers cool,
the thunder lilies bloom.

But there's something else.

And you don't have to pay much attention to notice it. You'll see it, smell it, and definitely hear it. It'll take you into its fold whether you like it or not. It's called the Wedding Season.

India's favourite season. As the austere Navratras come to a close, and good vanquishes evil, India gets ready to party like it is going out of fashion. A tsunami of a time that brings with it mazzedar parties, epic traffic jams, dancing, shopping frenzy, the thunder of dhols to keep you awake all night long, high heels the size of a building, barely there backless cholis, pretty fairy lights, and of course, those extra pounds after all the wedding food. What's not to love about it? It's festive, it's fun, and it's fabulous.

Band, Baajaa, Business

Nothing compares to the Indian wedding. Nothing at all. It's extravagance at its finest. It's such a big affair that the *Wall Street Journal* reported that on the evening of 27 November 2012 there were 60,000 weddings in Delhi and 1,00,000 in the entire month.[1] That's just one state. When you take into account the entire country— the maths can boggle the mind. I toh will get a headache just thinking of those numbers. But if you're the numbers kind of person and want proof, here's a *Business Today* snippet for you: 'San Francisco-based software development company Veristrat launched a wedding management software for India, called Shaadi-e-Khas, in

April 2011. CEO Bharat Kanodia pegs the size of the Indian wedding market—which includes all expenses incurred at a wedding—at about $25 billion, or Rs 1.25 lakh crore, and growing at 25 to 30 percent a year.'[2]

Shaadi Census!

India's population is around 1.25 billion.
An average Indian family has five members.
There are around 250 million families in India.
With about one marriage per family every 20 years, the country averages roughly 10 million marriages every year!

Gone are the days of laddoos and shehnais. Today, it's big bucks all the way. With destination weddings, designer saris and florists, theme weddings, performances by celebrities, and a baaraat that will give the opening ceremony of the IPL a run for their money. Arrey, we've even taken over a French palace and overrun it with elephants and dandia! You know what I mean, na? J

So much so that the Indian wedding season also drives up gold prices in the international markets. It's more than just the sangeets and cocktail parties and Tahiliani saris, ladies. With every kundan set bought, you too, are contributing to the economic tide of the country, albeit in a very fashionable and glitzy way.

But enough of all of this. We read about this stuff in the papers every year. What we tend to sometimes forget amid all this hoo-haa is the girl at the centre of it all. The reason behind the booming wedding industry and the ones getting fat on it. The girl at the threshold of womanhood. The Bride herself.

Bridezillas

'Godzilla has nothing on a bride-to-be planning her dream wedding . . .' We've all heard about or watched an episode of the supremely catchy show called *Bridezilla*. Isn't it sad that a beautiful ceremony celebrating the union between a man and woman has become so distorted and mad? I think it is. Like I said before, at the bottom of this big show is the classic keeping up with the Joneses. Today we earn more than we did a decade ago. Post-liberalization, the Indian economy boomed and our simple lifestyles were transformed forever. There is no going back to that simple life. The more we have, the more we want. And brides suffer the worst from it. The pressure to have the biggest, baddest wedding wears her thin. And I have women coming to me all the time to lose (sometimes a challenging number of kilos in a challenging period of time) weight before their weddings. Some girls I have counselled have horrifying stories of crash diets, quick fixes, diet pills, extreme exercise plans, and juicing programmes that do nothing but cause further health complications. Too many brides-to-be resort to extreme measures and quick fixes to drop the kilos in a hurry. Some of those methods may work a little (even if they're not so safe or healthy), but often times they fail—miserably. Because they aren't the right solutions or the right way of going about things.

I understand that everyone wants to look good on their wedding day but such drastic measures are definitely what you should not resort to.

My philosophy on being fit is really quite simple— you are what you eat. And if you follow a healthy regime on most days of the week, you're good as gold. Diets should only be resorted to when it's the last option. A healthy balanced diet is key to everything. For example: you don't wait till the last moment to work on the assignment your boss had given you a month ago. (Or do you?) Similarly, you shouldn't have to hurry and go on crash diets just before your wedding. A bit of planning can go a long way.

The best thing about a wedding is that it isn't going to happen tomorrow. It's a deadline that's generally in the near future. This means that you can plan towards it. You don't have to go crazy in the last week, which should be reserved for more relaxing things like visits to the parlour or a good night's sleep.

Why am I going on about this?

Because it's very very important. A diet can only work if you *enjoy* doing it, and give it the time it needs. As with everything natural, bodies don't change overnight. And crash diets are never fun. That's why I propose you start as early as you can. The fact that you know the date of the wedding makes life much simpler. Look at it as a positive.

Not Quite Hitched but Want to Get Fit Still?

Even for those of you who aren't getting married, but perhaps there's a big wedding coming up in the family, you can still use this date as a marker on your calendar for good health. Use this date as your end goal. Mark it up in bold and plan backwards. How many kilos before you reach your ideal weight? How much time will it take you to achieve that goal?

Keep in mind that losing weight isn't just a fashion statement. Gone are the days of size zero. Today, what you should aim for is reaching your ideal weight, which is NEVER a fixed number. Your ideal weight is always in a range. Aim for that. For example, if you're 30 years old and measure 5 feet 3 inches, your ideal weight is anywhere between 47 and 50. At your ideal weight, health complications come down drastically. In America, heart disease is the biggest killer, topping cancer and crime, and since we have more and more restaurants opening up in India coupled with growing affluence, a similar trend is visible here. We are replicating a lifestyle which is far from ideal or healthy. Obesity is rocketing in India. I know this because the number of clients I have increases every year, and each year, the weighing scales also see bigger figures.

Stay Motivated

Here are a few steps to keep your motivation up so that you feel energetic enough to follow through to your goal and keep on track.

1. **Analyse your history:** When a client comes to me, I make her/him tell me everything they've done or tried in the area of health and nutrition, their failures and their successes, what worked for them and what didn't. And when they start on my programme, the first thing they have to show me when they come for their visit is their food diary, where they must write everything they've eaten, and I mean *everything*—even if it's a handful of peanuts. This is so I can evaluate what's going on with their weight, why they're losing weight and why they aren't.

   An analysis of your weight loss history is important because then you know where you stand. You know what you can take and what you can't. This is my first advice to you, my dear readers—before you read any further, take 20 minutes out to do this. The first thing everyone should do before they make a commitment to start something new. Reflect on your past. Think back to the last few diets or weight loss experiments or workouts you've tried. What made you quit? Did they work? Did you achieve your goal? What part about it did you hate the most? Was it too lengthy a programme? Or too strict? Too strenuous? It's important that you write these down so you can evaluate what doesn't work for you. There is really no point if you keep trying things only to discard them. What you need is to find something that is tailored to your life that suits you, and most importantly, works for you. A simple pro–con list like the one below will work.

Diet plan	Workout programme	Weight lost or not	Pros	Cons
Detox Juicing	Yoga	3 kgs	Weight lost!	– Was hungry all the time – Felt faint –Will never do it again!!

2. **Identifying your goals and rewarding yourself:** After you've analysed your weight loss history, the next step is to identify the amount of weight you want to lose. Part II of the book has all the weight loss plans. Select the one that's relevant to you. For example, if you want to lose 4 kilos, then choose the upto 5 programme. Once you know your goal, I'll tell you how many months you need to lose that weight. And you'll be on your way to hotness!

3. **Rewarding yourself:** I know people who pretend tiresome things are a game to make it livelier. After all, when our day-to-day lives get monotonous, we go on holiday. Apply the same trick here since you can't go on a holiday from your diet plan otherwise it'll defeat the very purpose of it. Every time you drop a few kilos, reward yourself with something special, like a pedicure or spa day. This way the diet will seem like a fun activity instead of a boot camp.

4. **Exercise is non-negotiable:** No amount of dieting will work on its own. Pick a physical

activity that you enjoy doing. It could be anything from cycling to dancing to Pilates. Make time for it. Remember, the more you exercise, the more energy you will have, the easier it will be to stay focused. Take a moment to stop and analyse how a new workout or healthy recipe affected your body. Did you sleep better? How was your mood? Remind yourself of these positive changes if you start losing motivation.

Find a way to make exercise fun and you will keep the momentum. While completing your daily cardio, listen to your favourite music—you will be amazed at how much longer you can stay on the treadmill when your favourite TV show is on! Also, consider what type of exercises you are committing to and consider what types of exercise you most enjoy. And if you really hate all forms of physical activity, use the exercises provided in this book to complement your diet. They're easy, can be done in your bedroom, and you have no excuse to not try them.

5. **Don't lose sight of the big day**: Between wedding planning, a career and a variety of social commitments, it is easy to lose sight of the excitement surrounding your big day. Don't lose track of it. Imagine yourself in that gorgeous sari (that you're going to be paying a bomb for) to keep you on track. Find inspiration from visualizing that special moment and stay motivated. Don't lose sight of that wonderful picture!

11

Pivotal Moment

Now the time has finally come when you can re-evaluate what you want from yourself and others. Your wedding day is a momentous event. One that is going to take you on a different path in life. Along with this comes new freedom, responsibilities and a change in outlook. Even amid the stress of wedding planning, it is possible to stick with or even start a healthy diet and fitness programme and lose weight. How? Commit to your plan. You just have to choose to stay in control, one day at a time, no matter what life and wedding planners may throw at you. Use the time leading up to your wedding to think about and revaluate what your priorities are. You are beginning a new chapter of your life. A fresh start. So why not start this new slice of life by looking and feeling good and healthy. It's a great motivator—one that spurs you on to accomplish many things, including losing that extra bit of weight that has haunted you all your life.

Coming Up Next

Are you healthy?

How do you know if you are?

Are you eating right?

Questions, questions and more questions is all I've got from my clients in all these years. So the next chapter, appropriately, is a questionnaire that helps you evaluate where you stand in the health index. After all, there's nothing like a good question to spark off a chain of effective solutions.

2

Are You Bridelicious?

'I never go out unless I look like Joan Crawford the movie star.
If you want to see the girl next door, go next door'
—Joan Crawford

I always stress that you have to know where you stand before starting anything new. There is no point in diving headlong into any diet or nutrition programme before understanding your body type, your body's needs, your level of health and fitness, and what drives or motivates you. Otherwise, you'll just be going through the motions without knowledge or more dangerously—with little knowledge. But this is where I can help you get some clarity. Like I always say, there's nothing you can't change. And there's nothing like a little bit of change to motivate you. So let's get started. Answer these questions honestly and see where you stand and what you have to change to be bridelicious in no time.

1. **What is the first thing you drink in the morning?**
   a. Herbal tea
   b. Water
   c. Coffee

2. **Your breakfast is . . .**
   a. A sandwich from the office cafeteria
   b. Eggs, bread, fruit, juice, the works. I love breakfast!
   c. Who has time for breakfast?!

3. **You need to pop by the market to buy a few things. It's about a kilometre away, you . . .**
   a. Walk to an auto to take you there
   b. Walk, of course
   c. Drive

4. **How many times a week do you exercise?**
   a. Whenever I can find the time
   b. Five
   c. Never

5. **What is your BMI (Body Mass Index)*?**
   a. Under 18.5
   b. 18.5 to 24.9
   c. Over 25

* *Divide your body weight by your height squared. Then you times that by 703. BMI = Weight (lb) / (Height [in] x Height [in]) x 703. Your BMI is quite an accurate measurement to understand if you are overweight or not.*

6. Do you smoke?
- a. On occasion
- b. Never
- c. Yes

7. What do you usually do in the evening?
- a. Spend time with friends and family
- b. Go out to play or walk the dog
- c. Surf the Internet, go to the movies

8. How many hours of sleep do you get at night?
- a. 8 or more
- b. Around 6
- c. 4 or less

9. What time do you have dinner?
- a. 9-ish
- b. 7.30 to 8
- c. Ummm. 11?

10. If you're not doing any exercise, which of these best describes why?
- a. I'm too tired
- b. I don't have time
- c. It's hard work

11. What do you feel like after you climb a flight of stairs?
- a. Out of breath
- b. Generally okay
- c. Sorry. I take the elevator. Always.

12. How much water do you drink daily?
a. I drink whenever I'm thirsty
b. 3 litres
c. A glass or so. I don't keep count.

13. What kind of carbs are you eating?
a. A mix of whole wheat and simple carbs
b. Only complex carbs
c. Don't understand the difference

14. What are your thoughts about dairy?
a. I drink a glass of milk a day
b. I eat raita or plain curd with lunch and dinner
c. Cheese is one of my favourite foods

15. How do you go grocery shopping?
a. I go out and fetch supplies when I need them
b. I make a list and shop every Sunday
c. Grocery shopping is not really my thing. I order my groceries when I need them online or have them delivered

The Verdict

Mostly As
You're almost there but not quite. You're walking a fine line between being fit and unhealthy. But fear not. All is not lost! What you need is a slight push in the right direction and soon you'll be a glowing bride.

Start with the simple and healthy recipes in this book and include a steady exercise programme into your daily routine. You need to work on your muscle strength. Try doing exercises that use your body weight for resistance. Adults should do at least 150 minutes moderate or 75 minutes vigorous physical activity a week. Consider building activities into your daily routine, like walking more or cycling to get around.

Mostly Bs

You go, girl! You know what your body requires and already have a healthy and fit lifestyle. This book will help you to become even lovelier than you already are. Adapt the timetable and recipes I set out in this book into your daily routine to see great results. There are many recipes that involve oil-free cooking— you can definitely benefit from it. Some people find my early dinner rule rigid and difficult but it shouldn't be too difficult for you since you already eat quite early.

Mostly Cs

Based on your responses today you're not very active and struggling with motivation. You need to start with baby steps. You'll soon gain in confidence and feel better. But you need to start now. Your lifestyle is a product of our modern times, and I understand that it can be very difficult to break free from things that your friends may be doing or from trends. However, that said, your health and life is your own and you'll have no one else to blame later when the first problems start cropping up. But the beautiful thing about the human body is that it forgives, heals and adapts quickly.

It's very important that you start being more active to reduce your risk of heart disease, stroke and Type 1 diabetes. Try out lots of different activities to find something you can enjoy on a regular basis. Evidence shows that even shorter sessions of moderate to vigorous physical activity can be good for your health. Ten minutes or more is a great starting point if you're struggling with time or motivation.

To get you to be Bridelicious, I'm going to get you started on a programme that will not only help you shed those pounds quickly—you'll start seeing results in a week to ten days and that will motivate you to keep going.

Coming Up Next

The next chapter is the meat of the book. What we're going to discuss is eating correctly—how much, at what time and what foods. Be prepared to revise your notions on food.

3

The Beautiful Bride Programme

'The groom always smiles proudly because he's convinced he's
accomplished something quite wonderful. The bride smiles
because she's been able to convince him of it'
—**Judith McNaught**, *A Kingdom of Dreams*[1]

Mallika came to me when she was forty years old and
weighing a whopping 149 kilos. This was four years ago.
She was a successful businesswomen and an inspiring
interior designer. After my first counselling session with
her I found that strangely enough, she hadn't come to
me because she wanted to lose weight. She had grown
used to it, and her daily affairs kept her busy enough not
to give it much thought. It was her family, she told me,
who had given her the ultimatum. They were worried
senseless about her weight and were breathing down her
neck to undergo a painful and dangerous gastro-biopsy.
It was that which made her come and consult me. She
didn't want to undergo surgery. Who does?

I took her on, and asked her to get her medical tests done. Surprisingly, she had no medical issues.

Mallika started with a lot of hiccups—she didn't want to eat my food, and she had great difficulty exercising, due to her weight. It took about a month of hemming and hawing but eventually, she settled in. I started her out with some basic swimming and some mild exercises. After the first month she lost 5 kilos. This was her water weight due to water retention. The 5 shed kilos was her turning point. She was so excited by the loss, that she became tremendously motivated by the programme. Gradually, she moved on to gymming and brisk walking even. Her energy was fantastic—the best case I've seen in all my years.

Six months later, Mallika's weight was at a staggering 89 kilos. She was beginning to run, climb stairs much faster, and the best part of it all—her family got off her back about the surgery.

Mallika's story is an inspiration for everyone out there who wants to lose weight. If she could come down from 149 to 89 (and counting) what's stopping you from losing a few kilos? Brides-to-be, this is your chance to get inspired by Mallika's achievement. Keep her in mind, and plough through and you'll be looking as gorgeous on the night of your wedding as you should.

If you've read my first book *Lose a Kilo a Week,* then you'll be familiar with my philosophy and programme. But newbies, read on with care, as what I explain in this chapter is the core to losing weight and being healthy. **Everyone,**

not only brides, can benefit from this programme, because it outlines some basic and universal concepts about eating right and staying fit. Why this programme works is because my clients see RESULTS in just one or two weeks and that makes a world of a difference in the long run. Results results results. Yes, I'll shout it out from the top of a building if I have to. Nothing else gives people a boost to carry on doing anything but results. After all my years as a dietician, I've found that it is only this that makes people continue on a programme and seriously lose weight. Think about it like this: If you've bought a cream and after using it for a week or two your skin starts looking fabulous, would you continue using it or forget about it, letting it languish in your medicine cabinet? I think the answer will always be the same: continue using it because it's giving you positive results.

So what are these results? you may ask. If you follow the programme sincerely, here are the differences you will see and enjoy.

In the first 1 to 2 weeks:
- lose a few kilos
- skin will start to glow
- more energy to take on daily activities
- spring in your step
- stomach will go in
- increase in confidence
- better bowel movement
- mind will be clearer and less sluggish

From week 3 onwards:
- your clothes will not hug you
- hair will feel glossier
- nails will become stronger
- less flatulence in the mornings
- tongue will not have a white coat in the mornings
- a positive change in attitude and confidence
- you will have energy to pack in more things into a day's schedule

I want to be honest with you. In all my years as a dietician, I've seen some people succeed while others fail. What I've noticed about the ones who succeed is that they're sincere, hard-working and generally excited about the programme. And if you've signed up for something, like reading this book, I know that you're keen or curious about getting in shape. Which is always a good sign. This is the first step to getting back on the health track. And since you're reading this book now, I know you've taken the first step towards that success. I can help you if you let me. And once you see the results my programme can give you, I can assure you you'll keep coming back for more!

The 3 Cs
I will begin by talking about the 3 important Cs:
- Time Control
- Portion Control
- Mind Control (I've dedicated all of Chapter 4 to this point)

Let's begin with the first.

1. Time Control

No one can control time. Yet we can find a way to make sense of it. In our hectic and modern lives today, we are in time's iron grip—running like headless chickens from one task to another, going out, keeping up with our friends and relatives. We are a slave to time. And not in a good way. There was a time when people woke up early and went to bed early. Because they knew that's what made man healthy, wealthy and wise. Today, we've taken that treasured philosophy and flushed it down the toilet. There is another saying that makes a lot of sense— eat breakfast like a king, lunch like a prince and dinner like a pauper. But we've rubbished that too. Nowadays, we eat when and what we feel like, throwing all good advice to the wind.

But remember—time is key.

It is what this programme is centred on. It is the axis of this diet. Because once you've figured out how and why time works in losing weight, you'll never question its basis. And trust me when I say this, you'll cherish it for life.

Eating at the right time can solve 90 per cent of your weight problems.

Yes. Feel free to cut that out and stick it on your board. Time is the trick to losing weight. Let's begin with the basics.

Your Body's Alarm Clock

The body clock is one of the most important systems that govern our bodies. If we change it due to work schedules or other lifestyle issues, then we risk major physical problems. You must have felt irritable or grumpy if you get very little sleep. But did you know that sleep deprivation can lead to bigger problems because it has upset your entire circadian system?

Here are some of the problems caused by sleep deprivation:

- Heart disease
- Heart attack
- High blood pressure
- Diabetes
- Kills sex drive
- Ages your skin

Sleep and Skin

When you don't get enough sleep, your body releases more of the stress hormone cortisol. In excess amounts, cortisol can break down skin collagen, the protein that keeps skin smooth and elastic.

- Makes you forgetful
- Leads to depression
- Causes weight gain

Light and darkness govern the human body more than you think they do. The circadian system is a person's internal biological alarm clock, a variety of biological processes according to an approximate 24-hour period. The body systems with the most prominent circadian variations are the sleep–wake cycle, the temperature regulation system, the digestive system and the endocrine system. In human beings, the sleep–wake cycle system depends on light and temperature. Which means that the sun's position during the day activates your body clock. And your body clock affects your digestive and metabolic rate.

Eating with the Sun
This means, very simply, that we should wake and eat with the sun and sleep when it sets. The second part is quite impossible to do as our urban schedules will not allow it. But we can control the digestive part of it. So we should eat according to the sun's position during the day because our metabolic system works according to it.

Which means we should eat our first meal not long after waking up, timing it with sunrise. From sunrise to noon, our metabolic rate is at its highest. This is also the time of the day when we are at our busiest. So whatever you eat during this time will burn easily. After noon, our metabolic rate slows down. And as evening approaches, it slows down even further, almost grinding to a halt by night-time. By sunset, our body is not ready to receive any more food. This is the time when our body is processing the day's intake and readying for elimination the

25

next day. So it is only wise to stop eating and loading the body with extra work. Unfortunately, most people today do the opposite. They skip breakfast and eat a heavy dinner. And even if you think that by skipping breakfast and eating a healthy dinner, you are doing your body good, you're wrong. Because you're not following your body's ideal timetable that has been already set by the workings of light and darkness.

The *New York Times* did a fascinating report on how lack of sleep can make you put on weight.

'Large population studies show that both adults and children are more likely to be overweight and obese the less they sleep at night. In smaller, controlled studies, scientists find that when people are allowed to sleep eight hours one night and then half that amount on another, they end up eating more on the days when they've had less sleep.'[2]

And you think I harp on and on about how important it is to go to bed early.

Ideal Timetable

Here I'm going to set out your body's ideal timetable. If you are serious about losing weight, you must try very hard to stick to it. It is what your body wants and is begging you for.

- **5 to 6 a.m.:** As the sun rises, so does your body. It wakes up and gets your internal organs ready for elimination and for fresh nutrients and energy.

- **8 to 9 a.m.:** Your metabolic rate is working very fast during this time. Your body is asking you for energy supplies, so you need to give it as much of the good stuff as you can. Have a generous and healthy breakfast. This meal sets the tone for the rest of the day. Your breakfast should give you enough energy to sustain you till noon. So think lots of healthy carbs. Whatever you do, do not starve yourself during this time. Break the fast that your body has been on through the night.

Skipping Breakfast Can Make You Fat

Did you know that skipping this important meal can actually make you fat?

If you deprive your body of energy supplies during this time of the day, your body will go into survival mode and hold onto its fat reserves because it thinks it will not get any energy. It is a basic survival response but one that will not help you lose weight. Most overweight people tend to skip this crucial meal.

To stop this from happening, ensure that you have breakfast at a regular time every morning, and make it a good one.

- **Noon to 1 p.m.:** The sun is at its peak, and so is your body's metabolic rate. Your body needs energy and a healthy lunch. By now, your body has done the maximum work and is heading towards a slowdown. This is also a time when your body is burning calories much faster than later in the day. Give yourself energizing food consisting of carbs and hi-fibre items.

- **6 to 7 p.m.:** As the sun sets, so does your metabolic rate. Your body wraps up the burning process and the body's juices start the process of absorption and assimilation, preparing for the elimination process for the following morning. Try not to eat after sunset. Whatever you eat after this time will turn toxic, making your entire system slow and sluggish. I know that this is the most difficult part of the plan. Most of us in the cities still work past this hour and not eating after 7 p.m. seems like a cruel joke. But it has to be done if you want to lose weight. Once you get a hang of this habit, you'll be so amazed by the wonderful results it yields that it will become a habit for life. All my clients who have nurtured this habit have thanked me time and time again for this precious little gem of advice.

FOOD–TIME PYRAMID

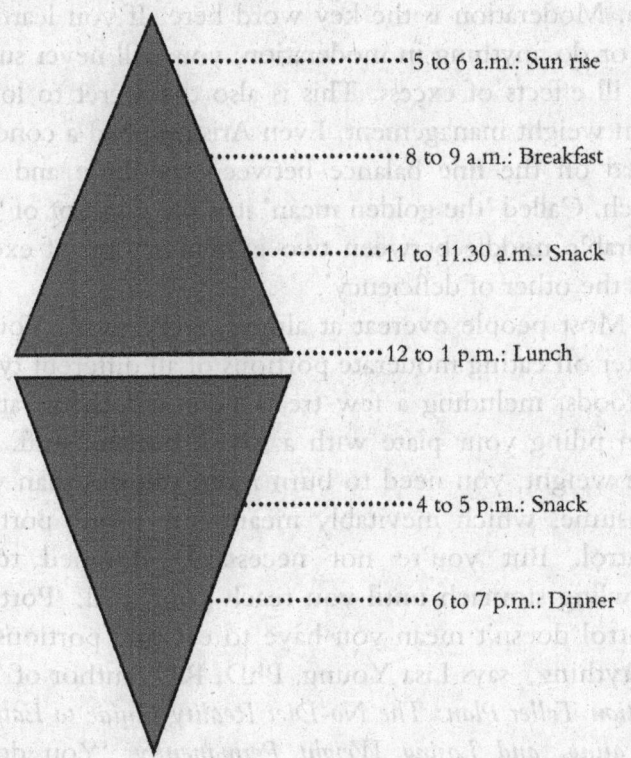

...... 5 to 6 a.m.: Sun rise

...... 8 to 9 a.m.: Breakfast

...... 11 to 11.30 a.m.: Snack

...... 12 to 1 p.m.: Lunch

...... 4 to 5 p.m.: Snack

...... 6 to 7 p.m.: Dinner

2. Portion Control

'Health is the natural condition. When sickness occurs, it is a sign that Nature has gone off course because of a physical or mental imbalance. The road to health for everyone is through moderation, harmony, and a "sound mind in a sound body".'—Jostein Gaarder, *Sophie's World*[5]

Portion control is all about knowing how much will satiate you and how much energy you need to sustain you. Moderation is the key word here. If you learn to eat or do anything in moderation, you will never suffer the ill effects of excess. This is also the secret to long-term weight management. Even Aristotle had a concept based on the fine balance between too little and too much. Called 'the golden mean' it is the concept of 'the desirable middle between two extremes, one of excess and the other of deficiency'.

Most people overeat at almost every meal. You're better off eating moderate portions of all different types of foods, including a few treats here and there rather than piling your plate with a lot of healthy stuff. To lose weight, you need to burn more calories than you consume, which inevitably means one thing: portion control. But you're not necessarily doomed to a growling stomach until you reach your goal. 'Portion control doesn't mean you have to eat tiny portions of everything,' says Lisa Young, PhD, RD, author of *The Portion Teller Plan: The No-Diet Reality Guide to Eating, Cheating, and Losing Weight Permanently*. 'You don't want to feel like you're on a diet, but you have to eat fewer calories.'[4]

Master your portions and you'll master your waistline.

But how, you'll ask me, do I tame this beast Moderation?

Here are a few time-tested secrets and tips to control your portions.

1. Before your meal, eat a salad

Filling up on fibre-and water-rich foods first can help prevent you from overdoing high-calorie fare later. A *Good Housekeeping* report details: 'In a study of 42 women at Penn State University, those who ate a big, low-cal salad consumed 12 percent less pasta afterward—even though they were offered as much as they wanted. The secret, say researchers, is the sheer volume of a salad, which makes you feel too full to pig out.'[5] Eat a salad 45 minutes to one hour before your main meal. This way you won't come to lunch or dinner starved and gorge on everything. Most salads have a few vegetables that have negative calories, which means it takes more energy to chew and digest them than you get from it. Also, raw or semi-raw foods are rich in fibre and will fill you up.

Salad wonder vegetables: Celery, cucumber, cabbage, iceberg, asparagus, lettuce, grapefruit, rocket leaves.

Grapefruit, We Love You!

'A 2006 study of 91 obese people conducted at the Nutrition and Metabolic Research Center at Scripps Clinic found that eating half a grapefruit before each meal or drinking a serving of the juice three times a day helped people drop more than three pounds over 12 weeks. The fruit's phytochemicals reduce insulin levels, a process that may force your body to convert calories into energy rather than flab.'[6]

Source: *Good Housekeeping*

2. Switch to green tea

In a recent Japanese study, 35 men who drank a bottle of oolong tea mixed with green tea catechins lost weight, boosted their metabolism, and had a significant drop in their BMI. In green tea, antioxidants called catechins are what help speed metabolism and burn fat.[7]

3. Keep your stomach half-full

This is every smart dieter's time-tested trick. By keeping your stomach half-full always, you will never feel the need to binge. Your stomach will be happy and never crave a huge meal.

How to achieve this?

You can easily master this trick by eating a few pieces of fruit every 20 to 30 minutes between your main meals. Cut up different types of fruit into small cubes and pack them in a handy tiffin. Put an alarm on your phone for every 20 to 30 minutes and on snooze after that. Do this till your main meal. You will never be famished because the fruit will ensure that your stomach is not completely empty, thereby avoiding the disastrous pig-out.

4. Smaller cutlery

Pick out smaller plates, bowls, cups and glassware in your kitchen and measure what they hold. You might find that a bowl you thought held 250 gm of soup actually holds 450, meaning you've been eating twice what you planned. Take control of your portions by downsizing your plate size. Switch from a regular dining plate to a quarter plate.

5. Eat slowly

It takes your stomach 20 minutes to register that the food has arrived and for you to start feeling the effects. If you eat fast, you just end up shovelling extra amounts of unwanted food into you. Take time to look at what you're eating. Look at its colour and savour the flavours and textures. Only then will eating be a wholesome experience. This will also mean that you'll eat slowly and less.

6. No second helpings

Take as much as you want in one go. Fill your plate with servings of vegetables and meat and carbs, but make sure you don't go back for more.

7. Include olive oil in your diet

Fight off middle-age pounds with extra virgin olive oil. A monounsaturated fat, it'll help you burn calories. It works just as well in salad dressings, as a bread dip, or for sautéing.

8. Measure oil carefully

This is especially important because oil (even the healthful kinds like olive and safflower) have so many calories; don't pour it directly into your cooking pan or over food.

9. Listen to your hunger cues

Eat when hungry and stop when satisfied or comfortably full. Try to gauge when you are 80 per cent full and stop there. Every meal is not your last.

The CCQ Diet

The ethos of my diet can be called CCQ in short. It means: low cal, low carb, low quantity.

I know a lot of people get put off by anything that limits their food intake. But you have to understand that **the only way to lose weight is by cutting down on your portions of carbohydrate, obviously supplemented by exercise**. Some people are able to lose a lot of weight this way without experiencing much hunger at all. Studies show that, under conditions of carbohydrate restriction, fuel sources shift from glucose and fatty acids to fatty acids and ketones, and that carbohydrate-restricted diets lead to appetite reduction and weight loss. **A low-carb approach to weight loss leads to automatic fat loss.** However, you can't cut it out completely. Those are great sources of energy and will help you really feel great and empowered while tackling your exercise programme. You need them. Plus, your will to exercise will be much greater, and your energy levels will be much higher if you maintain a healthy intake of carbs per day. Cutting them out will make you feel tired and constantly starved for food you can't have. A good, moderated amount of carbs will really help you burn calories and stay motivated to go to the gym.

The idea behind the diet is to cut down the food you're currently eating from a lot to a little less. What I'm going to focus on in this diet is to burn that fat with a combination of eating right and exercising. This diet is fashioned on simple mathematics. It's clear, logical and works like a dream. It's called a deficit calorie diet and works on cutting back the number of calories you consume in a day by a bit. The diet gives you less calories than you require in a day thereby burning your body's fat reserves to give you the required energy instead of it coming from food. The mind–stomach connection takes 20 minutes. So it takes 20 minutes for your brain to register that you are full. What you generally do is overstuff yourself in those 20 minutes. What I am going to do is make you stop eating when your stomach is half-full.

A Recap from *Lose a Kilo a Week.*

There are 3,500 calories in one pound (0.45 kilo, that is almost half a kilo) of body fat. The rule of thumb of my diet is creating an 'energy deficit' of 3,500 calories (equivalent to 1 pound of fat) in order to lose one pound.

So to lose one kilo in one week, you are going to focus on creating a deficit of 1000 calories a day, which over the course of one week will result in 1 kilo of weight loss (1000 calories x 7 days = 7,000 calories). Of course, the 1000 calories are not going to be cut out from food alone. It will be a combination of less food, therapy and exercise. By this logic, you can lose up to 4 kilos a month, and even more if you work hard.

*Remember that you will not be on a deficit calorie diet for the rest of your life. It's just till you get back to your natural weight. After you reach your ideal weight all you have to do is maintain that ideal weight.

The Formula of the Meal Plans

Here's the basic formula that you must learn. Make it your mantra and watch the pounds shed. You can use this skeleton and adapt it to suit your palate and foods that you enjoy.

As you go along you'll notice that all the meal plans follow a formula. They are a perfect combination of carbs, fibre and protein. If you ever get lost along the way and want to remember what constitutes a balanced meal, return to this box. Here I'll give you a simple formula to help you plan out your own meal.

Breakfast

Calcium + Carb + Protein
(Skimmed milk + multigrain bread or oats + egg white)

Mid-morning Snack

Negative calories
(Green salad without dressing)

Lunch

Carbs + Fibre + Calcium
(Wholegrain roti or rice + vegetables + curd)

Mid-afternoon Snack

Nibbles!
(Green tea + multigrain biscuits)

Dinner

Low carb + Low quantity + Low calories
(Clear soup + steamed veggies or boiled chicken)

To recap, what you need to keep in mind is what time you're eating your meals and that whatever you're having should be low carb, low quantity and low calories. It's the only way to lose weight. Be mindful of what goes into your mouth, even if it's a handful of peanuts. Once you recognize and learn to be watchful of what you're consuming, the road to fitness will even itself reach out for you.

Coming Up Next

Ever wanted to say no to something, but the word that came out of your mouth was an enthusiastic yes instead? Most of us fall prey to peer and family pressure and find ourselves tongue-tied when we have to reject something. In the next chapter, we'll discuss this tricky subject at length and I'll arm you with the tools of saying no to temptation without incurring anyone's wrath and displeasure.

4

'I Do . . . Not'
—Learning to Say No

'Self-knowledge is better than self-control any day,'
Raquel said firmly.
'And I know myself well enough to know how
I act around cookies.'
—**Claudia Gray**, *Evernight*[1]

The Science of Pleasure

Oscar Wilde once wrote: 'I can resist anything except temptation.' Good ole Wilde was right in more ways than we can imagine. Because how many of us can actually say no to temptation?

What if I told you that you can dilute its power and make it fade away?

The truth is that we can. It's called rewiring how we perceive food.

The human brain has a pleasure centre that works on the reward principle or the reward circuit. In simple terms, it means that if you like something, the pleasure centre of the brain will make a note of it and will reinforce the desire to perform the same pleasurable action again and again and again. Like listening to your favourite song on loop. Like overeating.

A person who overeats activates the same brain circuits as do behaviours linked to survival, such as bonding and sex. The food causes a surge in levels of a brain chemical called dopamine, the happiness hormone, which results in feelings of pleasure. The brain remembers this pleasure and wants it repeated. This is the case in most addiction-related issues. Food and, you'll be shocked, drugs and smoking too. In fact, research on addiction over the years has come to this fact—obese adults who binge on dense carbs and who are neither alcoholic nor drug-addicted have the same D2 dopamine gene marker that distinguishes alcoholism and other drug addictions. If you'd like to further read on this subject, I suggest you pick up neuroscientist David Linden's book *The Compass of Pleasure: How Our Brains Make Fatty Foods, Orgasm, Exercise, Marijuana, Generosity, Vodka, Learning, and Gambling Feel So Good*. In it, he traces the origins of pleasure in the human brain and how and why we become addicted to certain food, chemicals and behaviours.

Why am I going on about this? It's because understanding this makes the task of recognizing temptation for what it is.

It isn't you.

Temptation is a tough beast to slay, because it's more of an evolutionary survival programming. How are you going to fight the pleasure centre archives of your brain?

I have two answers:

1. Avoidance
2. Positive reinforcement

1. Avoidance

The first answer complements the second. One without the other is no fun. So how do you stay away from temptation?

I'm not asking you to hide out in a cave or under a rock till the storm of temptation passes. That's impossible to do. Temptation surrounds us in every form and every moment of life. What I suggest is staying away from the storm. It's just a change of POV, but it works.

Start out by changing how you shop. Look carefully at your grocery list. Do you really need double cream? And the chips? Who is going to eat it when you're the only one in the house all day? Who is going to come back hungry from office and reach for that packet? If the answer is you, you know what to do. It's really that simple—if something isn't within arm's reach, you'll think twice about stepping out of the house and going and buying it. De-addiction programmes use the same philosophy. If there are no cigarettes around then what is a smoker going to smoke? Nothing.

The next idea is the old switcheroo. It means to ditch and replace. Clean out your larder and fridge. Ditch all the food that is not on your diet. This doesn't mean you have an empty kitchen. Replace every unhealthy, taunting and high-calorie food item with something healthier. The next time hunger strikes, you'll be eating a granola bar instead of a chocolate one.

Eat before you step out. Hunger strikes at the most unlikeliest of places, and if your stomach is empty you're going to step up to the next chaatwalla and go berserk.

Recognize your hunger patterns. If you know you get hungry around 5 p.m., then keep a snack handy. An apple and a glass of water will do the trick. Most times, we feel a false sense of hunger. This happens when you're dehydrated. The next time your stomach is grumbling, try having a glass of water and see if you're really hungry or not.

2. Positive Reinforcement

'Positive reinforcement is the most important and most widely applied principle of behaviour analysis'—Cooper, Heron and Heward (2007).[2]

This is one of the most widely used methods of behaviour analysis and correction in the field of psychology. The same principles are used in the training of animals too. Remember the clicker and treat trick to get your dog to shake? It's quite like that but it isn't just for animal training—you train yourself and others every day in the methods of positive reinforcement, even without realizing it. For example, do you remember your parents promising you a present if you did excellently at your Class 12 examinations? That there was positive reinforcement. It's training a behaviour. It's pushing you to work harder so that you get your present at the end of it all. Positive reinforcement is the most pleasant and effective training method.

If temptation is grinding you thin, remind yourself of your goal, the benefits that come with it, and how good you'll feel when you achieve it. The next time you want food to make you feel happy, switch it with something else that gives you pleasure. If you like dancing, go out dancing! It can be anything that makes you happy. Your brain will start prioritizing this pleasure habit over food, giving it more prominence in its archives. The more you do it, the more inclined you will be towards activating your pleasure centre, the less importance food will play in this region, and this, in turn, will help you stay off food. You'll be rewiring your brain if you keep at it. Like I said before, it's not you but a tiny part of your brain that controls these habits. If you can tame that little beast, you're golden. But nothing comes without some old-fashioned determination. So think fit, think hot, and in some time, your brain will come to accept that as a pleasure instead of stuffing your face. Remember, if you think you can do it, you're damn right you can. Keep at it, with the knowledge that that there's a present waiting for you at the end of the journey.

Food-pushers

Image this.

You're in your masi's neighbourhood, and you drop in for a quick hello (heaven forbid she finds out that you were in the colony and didn't visit!). The 'quick hello' extends, as things generally do in this country, and soon chai is brought out. But it's never just chai is it? Chai, that innocent beverage, in Indian homes masquerades as one big spread—samosas, cookies, bhujia, cake—the works. You don't want to offend your masi, so you take a quick nibble of the cake—it's from Elma's and it's delicious, and very soon you're two slices down, and forgetting your diet faster than you can say Shahrukh Khan.

Was it very hard to imagine? I'm going to go with my guess, which is a resounding no!

Each and every one of us has been in this situation. If it isn't 'chai' then it's dealing with food-pushing relatives who will shovel food down your gullet, fattening you up for God knows what. And come the holidays or worse still, a wedding, the food pushing only gets worse. In India, especially, where saying 'no' to offered food is akin to committing a crime, how does one stay on track?

Food-pushers are generally well-meaning people. They probably aren't deliberately sabotaging you, so take a minute to help them understand your needs. But there comes a time when you have to say no, because food-pushers are difficult to avoid and almost impossible to refuse. You have to do it for the sake of looking hot and glamorous on your big day at least.

Here are some of the things you can do to keep food-pushers at arm's length and your kilograms in check.

1. **Honesty is actually the best policy:** Go out guns blazing! Tell your friends and family of your goals, how you need to lose X number of kilos, why you're doing it, how it's going to benefit you, and them too (if they give it a try). Tell them how difficult the road is, how you would love their support, etc. etc. Once you've put all your cards on the table, it'll be ridiculous and extremely insensitive if people still try and force-feed you! It's generally the best way to go about things.

2. **Actually saying no:** Saying no is always tough. The best of us are sometimes incapable of doing so. But keep your goal in mind and stick with it. The best way to say no is *how* you say it. Start with compliments. A bunch of them. Flattery will throw most people off. And then slip in your no—and do it with conviction and a smile. In a nutshell—be kind but firm.

3. **Reminding yourself:** Sometimes you have to say no to yourself. When the temptation is too great, remember that food isn't the only way to celebrate. Think of the other activities that motivate you or make you happy. It could be anything, like shopping for example, to take your mind off the nibbles.

4. **Arriving at an unwelcome hour:** If being honest and open doesn't work, then you have to take to

some underhand tactics. Nothing devious. But if you want to be hot and fit on D-Day, then nothing should stop you from reaching your goal, especially if you're trying your best. It's cheeky and sometimes in bad form to show up unannounced, but it's a trick to catch food-pushing relatives unawares. The chances of them cooking or ordering a spread are higher if they know you're visiting. So . . . Boo!

5. **Second helpings**: The quickest way out of second helpings is by using the marvellous tool of past tense. Try saying: 'Oh I absolutely loved the pasta, and I ate so much of it, that I won't have room for dessert. What went into it by the way?' Diversion is another time-tested dieter's trick.

6. **At parties**: Pre-wedding parties will come like a storm, with everyone inviting you over for drinks and food. Eat at home and then step out. Not the most favourable option but you'll be full already, and to resist bursting out of your dress, you'll automatically resist those calorie-laden canapés!

Bridal Invites, Parties and the Bachelorette

The lead up to weddings is a time for celebration. Naturally, you'll be invited to many parties, lunches, brunches, teas by friends and family who want to indulge you before the big day. But what about those calories that come along with it? On one hand, you're desperately trying to get fit and on the other, the cakes are not really helping you with your struggle. Let's face it, you can't avoid these situations and more importantly, you shouldn't have to. It's your wedding after all! The best way to *try* (key word here) and keep healthy AND have a good time is by choosing your food and drinks carefully.

To make it simple, I'm giving you a list of party food options that you must absolutely avoid and the ones that you can take a nibble of.

Absolute No No	Can Nibble
Indian	**Indian**
Rumali rotis Naans Missi rotis	Tandoori rotis
Pulao, biryani	Steamed rice
Any curry	Dry mixed vegetables
Matar paneer	Tandoori paneer
Kadhai chicken	Tandoori chicken
Dahi bhalla	Any raita without the bhalla
Black daals	A little bit of yellow daal
Continental/Chinese/World Cuisine	**Continental/Chinese/World Cuisine**
White-sauced-based pastas, etc.	Red-sauce-based pasta, chicken, etc.
Cream-based soups	Clear soups
Pad thai	Soupy ramens
Nachos, burritos, tacos, enchiladas	Salsa, burrito in a bowl without the tortilla wrap
Fried rice	Steamed rice
Curried dishes	Grilled, steamed or baked dishes

Absolute No No	Can Nibble
Continental/Chinese/World Cuisine	Continental/Chinese/World Cuisine
Peanut sauce	Teppanyaki
California rolls with heavy dressings	Sushi, sashimi
Spring rolls	Satay
Oyster sauce, hoisin sauce	Light soy sauce
Chopsuey	Steamed noodles (buckwheat like soba or udon noodles)
Red meat	Fish or chicken
Cream or milk-based desserts	Fruity desserts

With knowledge comes responsibility. Now that you know how your brain is wired and what you can do to stave off temptation, you should start acting on it immediately. Before you progress to the next few chapters, which deal with the actual programme and the diet, I want you to first go and clean out your larder and redo your grocery list. Once you've stocked up on healthy options, then continue reading. Happy spring-cleaning!

Coming Up Next

We're almost there, dear readers. The next part outlines diet plans and I've added many delicious and nutritious recipes that you can use in your diet. The next part is practical and gets down to the doing of it. So best of luck on your journey to good health!

PART II

Diet Plans and Oil-free Recipes

5

The Wedding Planner—
Getting Started

'A goal without a plan is just a wish'—**Antoine de Saint-Exupéry**

As with everything else in life, we need a plan, sometimes a very detailed one, to succeed or to just get by. I cannot emphasize this enough. Most times, we plan our work lives down to the detail—worksheets, trackers, schedules—yet we let our personal lives languish, procrastinating daily to achieve small goals. But one thing I have to acknowledge here, there's no better organizer than a bride. If you watch a bride go about her wedding plans, I have one simple advice for you—get out of her way! She'll put a general to shame. Juggling shopping dates with her army of friends and relatives, pandal arrangements, choosing the right caterers, menus, flower arrangements, lighting, etc. Planning an Indian wedding is a gargantuan task. So much so that today

51

most people just hire wedding planners to tackle the event. Amid this flurry of activities, most brides forget to plan one tiny and important part.

So here's my question: How many of you ladies or brides-to-be are planning out your daily nutrition and health aspects?

Most brides come to me at the eleventh hour. 'Nishi, help!' they'll call me frantically, 'I need to lose 5 kilos by next week. How do I do it?'

What can I say, ladies? I can do many things. I can also help you lose weight dramatically in a short period of time, but I'm no jaadugar, na? But it's essentially what all women are like. They get caught up in the big picture and forget to pay attention to themselves. I understand that sometimes we can't plan everything all the time. Then we wouldn't be human but like those *Transformers*. Hain na? But if it's something that is set in stone—like your wedding day—then there are no excuses for not planning a few months ahead. So that come D-Day and you'll look every bit ravishing as you should. There's really no point of the wedding looking better than you right. This is where I come in. In this chapter, I will help you outline a programme to lose those extra kilos and get you looking fit and healthy by the time you say 'I do'.

Getting Started: The 5-step Kick Start

Have you ever sat on a motorcycle? If you have, or seen one being started, you know that sometimes it takes a few good kicks to get it started. After which it is smooth sailing (or not!). Most diet plans are like kick starting a motorcycle. A few coughing starts, failures, but when you finally hit the right note, there's no looking back. Very often in life we fail to achieve our goals because we jump into them headlong without a thought or a plan, because we're impatient or just too excited to begin. The trick to actually achieving what we set out to do, is to take a moment before the adventure begins and think out the kinks and hurdles that will come in the journey. If we do our homework and research well, we would have done 50 per cent of the work. The rest is just application. Here's why I urge you to follow these 5-step kick starts. This preparation is important because I want you to succeed in this journey to good health. Once you've done the background work, it'll be much easier to work on the diet plans, rather than jumping into a big confusion ball, getting tired, bored or frightened of the plan, and giving up. So what are you waiting for—let's have a look at the five steps.

1. **Identifying your goal and problem areas:** As I mentioned before, the first thing you need to do is estimate how many kilos you need to lose. Think about the weight you were most comfortable in. The number that doesn't make you tired. The ideal number at which your health complications reduce, and at which you feel you have the energy to tackle each day without batting an eyelid. And *size zero* is not a goal. The BMI is a good calculator for your ideal weight but it doesn't take into consideration

many factors such as a person's waist, chest and hip measurements. It also doesn't consider bone density. But it is at best a basic indicator to where you stand weight-wise. Consult your doctor, if you don't know what your ideal weight should be.

After this, select the diet plan that suits you best. In this section, I have three broad diet plans. Diet Plan #1 is for those of you who want to lose up to 5 kilos. Diet Plan #2 is for those of you who want to lose between 5 to 10 kilos. And lastly, Diet Plan #3 is for those of you who want to lose anywhere between 10 and 20 kilos. Follow the plan made for you sincerely, and watch as the kilos shed away from you like warm clothes in summer.

Complement the diet with the exercises given in this book. Everyone has a problem area, be it the bum or the arms, or that tummy that just doesn't become blackboard flat no matter how many sit-ups you do. Although I recommend a holistic exercise programme for maximum impact, you can also choose to pick only those workouts that tackle your problem area.

2. **Doctor's check-up:** Vital, ladies. This is absolutely vital before you begin any diet or workout programme. We can never thoroughly be aware of the tiny, immaculate workings of our bodies. And we're not supposed to either. They're complex, finely balanced mechanisms that keep us alive and ticking. But it's very important to do a few tests before embarking on the journey. The most common reason for weight gain is an imbalance of hormones or the malfunctioning of a

vital organ. Your doctor will recommend a few basic tests to check if everything is in order.

A few things to check:

- Blood pressure
- Blood sugar
- Hormone tests such as TSH and FSH
- Complete blood count
- Liver tests

You also need to check if you're okay to start a workout programme. I've seen many people injure themselves by dashing into a workout that's too intensive for them. Be wary of such things. Always start slow and build up intensity to avoid severe injuries that can cause complications later on.

3. **The actual planning:** Once you've got the green signal from the doctor to start the Diet Plan, check with the Diet Plan that's appropriate for you to see how many days you need to achieve your goal. Calculate backwards from your wedding date. If you feel you need more time then you'll need to perhaps up the tempo.

4. **Setting aside time each day:** Make a timetable for yourself. Put down your daily chores and activities—everything that takes up any amount of time on your day-to-day schedule. Look at it closely and see where there is time for you to prepare and pack your lunches and snacks. You'll be doing a lot of that in the Diet Plans.

Mark out each free slot—that is when you'll be dedicating time to this diet. Also, mark out any other available free time—this is for your workout routine. Although early mornings and evenings are best to workout, if you're a super busy bee with a hectic schedule, grab any free time to prepare your food and workout. Beggars cannot be choosers! If you look closely at your schedule, you'll find that there are pockets of time waiting to be used. I've drawn up a rough schedule for what it can look like, but go ahead and make your own.

Time	What I'm generally up to	Free time!
7 a.m.	Wake up	
		Free time to workout AND pack a snack!
7.30 a.m.	Shower	
8 a.m.	Breakfast	
8.30 a.m.	Catch the metro!	
9 a.m.	Office	
6.30 p.m.	Back home	
		Free time to workout!
Up to 8 p.m.	Watch TV or go out with friends	
10 p.m.	Dinner	
		Free time to pack tomorrow's lunch!
Upto 1 a.m.	Surf the Internet, watch *Breaking Bad*	

5. **Stocking up:** After you've figured out your schedule
    and planned out how you're going to make this diet
    a part of your daily life, it's time to go shopping! This
    is the fun part. Refer to Chapter 4 (see p 42) about
    spring-cleaning your larder. Before you begin the
    diet I want you to remove all junk and processed
    food from your kitchen and fridge. Yes, even the
    chocolate, ladies. **Remember if you don't have
    it, you won't eat it!** Apart from your regular daals
    and veggies, load up on these foods:

Diet Plan Grocery List

Vegetables

- All leafy green veggies
- Carrots
- Peas
- Beetroot
- Cauliflower, cabbage, broccoli
- No potatoes, arvi, sweet potatoes, no cooked beetroot, yams.

Fruits

- Granny Smith apples
- Golden Shimla apples
- Kashmiri apples
- Mausambi
- Pomelo

- Guava
- Kiwi
- Strawberries
- Gooseberries
- No mangoes, custard apple, papaya, litchis, figs, watermelon, chikoo, pineapples

Grains

- Whole grains only like bajra, millet, quinoa, barley, ragi, amaranth, brown rice, whole wheat, rye, barley

No daals, red meat, egg yolks, white breads, rice or processed flour.

6. **Committing:** We're almost there, my lovely reader. Now for the last but equally important step. 'I'm going to start working out'; 'I'm going to travel more'; 'I'm going to buy a house'; 'I'm going to find the perfect guy'; 'I'm going to lose 15 kilos'; 'I'm going to stop smoking'.

   Sounds familiar?

   We all make new year resolutions. Only to break them a week later. After all, we're only human. There's only so much we can change about ourselves. That's why most new year resolutions don't hold up for very long—because we ask ourselves to change too many things, and most of them are unrealistic.

On the other hand, a Diet Plan like this, which is well formulated, well planned out and, most important, reasonable, is not a wishy washy daydream. If you follow these sincerely, it will guarantee results. But committing to anything is a tough job. It requires patience and determination. Strength and grit. That's why I suggest you bring in someone else into this journey. Tell your best friend or your parents what you are embarking on, involve them, tell them how much this goal means to you. Ask them for help. If they, too, want to lose weight, bring them in on it. There's nothing like working together towards something. You'll feel motivated when you see someone else doing it, even if it's just their support and not participation. You're more likely to succeed if you have a team cheering for you than going at it all by yourself. Most smokers who try to quit usually seek the support from the people who surround them. That way they can't slip easily under the watchful vigilance and care of their loved ones.

So go ahead, and tell your friends and family. Really, go shout it from the mountains!

Coming Up Next

The next chapter is the first Diet Plan for those of you who want to lose up to 5 kilos before the big day. I've included the diet charts—these are ideal plans but can be tweaked to suit your palate.

6

Diet Plan #1: Losing Up to 5 Kilos

'I am a better person when I have less on my plate'
—**Elizabeth Gilbert**, *Eat, Pray, Love*

Goal: Lose up to 5 kilos
Duration: 4 to 6 weeks

Now that we're done with all our prep work, shopping and planning, it's time to jump in!

This plan is for those of you who want to lose up to 5 kilos. The plan spans between 4 to 6 weeks. I always keep it at this range, because no two bodies are the same. And no two bodies will lose weight at the same rate. Some of us also won't follow the programme as strictly (we're all human, after all), so this time frame is what works best to lose this amount of weight.

Drink as much water as possible to keep hydrated through the programme. You need 1 litre of water a day for every 10 kg that you weigh.

The plans outlined are a skeleton or a base for you to expand on. Be creative. Remember to make this YOUR plan, so take cues from it and adapt it to suit your palate—as long as it isn't high-calorie food stuff! Use the oil-free recipes provided in this book to explore further into the art of low-calorie, delicious and nutritious meals.

Losing up to 5 kilos is not going to be difficult. You just need to work hard enough, stay off the processed food, and eat like I've taught you, and you're going to be slipping into that bodycon dress in no time. Without a hint of a bulge! So let's get you started!

A Note on the Diet Charts

Below are three examples of ideal meal plans. You will get maximum benefits if you adhere to the plans outlined. However, these plans are a skeleton of what your meals should be like, and you can adapt and tweak them to best suit your palate. This doesn't mean that you switch wholesome foods for chocolate and deep-fried items! Try to eat your meals as close to the given time as possible, otherwise it defeats the purpose of the diet. If your meal timings are drastically different from what I've outlined, take baby steps—gradually bring your eating time to match what I've given. The most important factor for success is timing, so you need to work on that first. Once you've managed to meet that requirement, then turn your concentration to the food part. Most importantly, have fun doing this! Bon appétit!

MEAL PLAN 1

Time	Food
On rising 7–7.30 a.m.	Hot water with lemon juice and ½ tsp of organic honey + Aloe vera juice (dilute 1 tsp of juice in a glass of water) + Tea/green tea (optional) (2 tsp skimmed milk, no sugar) + 5 almonds (soaked overnight)
Breakfast between 8 and 8.30 a.m.	Skimmed milk (100 ml) + Toast (oatmeal bread) with some sugar-free jam or green chutney
9.30–10 a.m.	½ orange
11–11.30 a.m.	Green salad with salt and lemon juice (no dressing)
Lunch between 12–12.30 p.m.	2 small rotis (oat flour + oat bran: 1 tbsp each) + Oil-free vegetables (avoid corn and potato) + Dahi/paneer (made with 150 ml milk)
1.30 p.m.	3–4 raspberries
3 p.m.	Green tea/regular tea (with 2 tsp of skimmed milk) + 2 oat biscuits
4.30 p.m.	2 strawberries

Time	Food
5. 30 p.m.	Salad/clear vegetable soup
6–6.30 p.m.	2 toasts (oat bread)
	+
	1 egg white
	+
	Salad

MEAL PLAN 2

Time	Food
On rising 7–7.30 a.m.	Hot water with lemon juice and ½ tsp of organic honey
	+
	Aloe vera juice (1 tsp diluted in a glass of water)
	+
	Green tea/regular tea
	(1 tsp skimmed milk, no sugar)
	+
	5 almonds
	(soaked overnight)
Breakfast between 8 and 8.30 a.m.	Milk (100 ml)
	+
	Oat flakes/oat bites (30 gms)
9.30–10 a.m.	½ piece of fruit
11.30 a.m.	Mixed green salad
	(avoid any heavy dressings)

Time	Food
Lunch between 12.30 to 1 p.m.	Brown rice (1 cup cooked rice) With oil-free vegetables (avoid potato and corn) or 1 chapati (barley + oat bran atta: 1 tbsp each) with oil-free vegetables (avoid potato and corn) + ½ cup of dahi
2 p.m.	½ piece of fruit
3–3.30 p.m.	Green tea/regular tea (2 tsp skimmed milk, no sugar) + 1 rye cracker with hung curd/green chutney
4.30 p.m.	½ piece of fruit
6 p.m.	Clear vegetable soup with ½ chicken breast + 1 slice toast (rye bread)

MEAL PLAN 3

Time	Food
On rising 7 a.m.	Aloe vera juice (1 tsp diluted in one glass of water) + Fresh amla juice (squeeze the juice of 1 amla) + Warm water with 1 tsp of flax seeds powder + Green tea/black coffee + 1 fig (soaked overnight)

The Bridal Diet

Time	Food
Breakfast between 8 and 8.30 a.m.	Soya milk (100 ml) + 1 roasted khakra or 2 besan idlis (made with 1 tbsp besan) with green chutney
9–9.30 a.m.	2–3 carrot sticks
10. 30 a.m.	¼ piece of orange
11–11.30 a.m.	Mixed salad (raw) with no dressing, lemon juice, salt and pepper
Lunch between 12 to 12.30 p.m.	Quinoa atta roti mixed with oat bran (1 tbsp each) with Oil-free vegetables (avoid potato and corn) and green chutney or Quinoa dalia with oil-free vegetables (avoid potato and corn) + Green chutney
2 p.m.	¼ sweet lime
3–3.30 p.m.	Tea/green tea/lemon water + A fistful of roasted channas
5.30 p.m.	Mixed homemade vegetable soup (200 ml)
6 p.m.	2 egg whites scrambled with vegetables (onions, tomatoes, mushrooms) or Steamed white fish (60 grams): sole, surmai, bassa + 1 bowl of steamed vegetables

Coming Up Next

The next chapter is the first Diet Plan for those of you who want to lose up to 10 kilos before your wedding day.

7

Diet Plan #2: Losing between 5 and 10 Kilos

'Nothing tastes as good as being thin feels'—
Elizabeth Berg, *The Day I Ate Whatever I Wanted:
and Other Small Acts of Liberation*

**Goal: Lose between 5 and 10 kilos
Duration: 8 to 13 weeks**

A Note on the Diet Charts

This is a much longer Diet Plan tailored for those of you who have more kilos to shed. And because the goal is bigger, I've spaced this out over a two- to three-month-long period. This gives you ample time to ease into the programme, to make it part of your life, and to see the results of it too.

Exercise is going to be vital for you in your goal to losing the kilos. A 20- to 30-minute workout every day will really give your diet a turbo boost. Keep the exercise simple but strenuous enough.

Drink a lot of water. Not drinking enough water is another cause of water retention. The body holds onto water, and if you're not drinking enough water, it'll hold onto whatever is already in.

The real gain of weight loss isn't just about fitting into your dream dress. It's far more serious than that. Every time you feel like giving up keep this in mind:

The Real Gains of Weight Loss

- Lower chances of heart attack or stroke
- Lowers risk of other heart diseases
- Lowers risk of Type 1 diabetes
- Lowers risk of certain types of cancer
- Lowers risk of infertility
- Lowers depression
- Lowers back pain and other back-related problems
- Increases life expectancy

MEAL PLAN 1

Time	Food
On rising 7 a.m.	Aloe vera juice (dilute 1 tsp of juice in a glass of water) + Fresh amla juice + ¼ tsp mix of flax, pumpkin, melon, watermelon, cucumber and papaya seeds + Tea/green tea (optional) (2 tsp skimmed milk, no sugar)
Breakfast between 8 and 8.30 a.m.	Oats upma (30 gms) with green chutney
9.30–10 a.m.	½ green apple
11–11.30 a.m.	Raw green salad with salt and lime
Lunch between 12.30–1 p.m.	Quinoa dalia (20 gms) with vegetables and green chutney
1.30–2 p.m.	2–3 raspberries
3–3.30 p.m.	Tea/green tea/coffee/lemon water + Roasted soya nuts (1 tbsp) or ½ cup curd with 1 strawberry
4.30–5 p.m.	¼ piece of fruit
5.30–6 p.m.	1 slice toast (rye bread) + 2 egg whites and salad

MEAL PLAN 2

Time	Food
On rising 7 a.m.	30 ml fresh wheat grass juice diluted in a glass of water + Aloe vera juice (1 tsp diluted in a glass of water) + ¼ tsp mix of flax, pumpkin, papaya seeds etc. + Green tea/regular tea (2 tsp skimmed milk, no sugar) + 3 almonds (soaked overnight)
Breakfast between 8 and 8.30 a.m.	Soy milk with ½ Weetabix
9.30–10 a.m.	¼ piece of fruit
11–11.30 a.m.	Mixed raw salad (avoid any heavy dressings)
Lunch between 12.30 to 1 p.m.	Brown rice (1 cup cooked rice) with ½ cup of any yellow dal or 1 chapati (barley + oat bran atta) with oil-free vegetables (avoid potato and corn)
2 p.m.	2 strawberries
3 p.m.	Green tea/regular tea/coffee (2 tsp skimmed milk, no sugar) + 1 oat biscuit
4–4.30 p.m.	¼ piece of green apple

Time	Food
5.30–6 p.m.	Toast or oat bread + 2 egg whites (scrambled) + Oil-free vegetables (avoid potato and corn) or Steamed white fish (60 gms) + 1 bowl of steamed/grilled vegetables

MEAL PLAN 3

Time	Food
On rising 7 a.m.	30 ml fresh wheat grass juice diluted in a glass of water + 1 tsp aloe vera juice diluted in one glass of water + ½ tsp flax seeds powder + ½ tsp of mixed seeds or Green tea/regular tea (2 tsp skimmed milk, no sugar) + 1 fig (soaked overnight)
Breakfast between 8 and 8.30 a.m.	Poha (brown flattened rice) + Vegetables with green chutney
11–11.30 a.m.	¼ piece of fruit

Time	Food
Lunch between 12 to 12.30 p.m.	1 roti made of kala channa atta + besan + oat bran (⅓ proportion of each) + ½ katori dahi (homemade skimmed milk)
2 p.m.	2–3 raspberries
3.30 p.m.	Soy milk (100 ml) or 1 boiled egg white
5 p.m.	¼ piece of guava
5.30–6 p.m.	Grilled/steamed chicken + 1 bowl of steamed vegetables or Tofu (60 gms) + Steamed vegetables

8

Diet Plan #3: Losing between 10 and 20 Kilos

'She'd even violated the only sensible rule of dieting she'd ever run across, the sage advice of the Muppets' Miss Piggy, who recommended never eating anything bigger than your head'—
Susan Donovan, *He Loves Lucy*

Goal: Lose between 10 and 20 kilos
Duration: 16 to 24 weeks

It was another hectic day at my previous clinic, Vasudevan's, in Greater Kailash, when one of the attendants told me that there was a lady waiting to see me. She didn't have an appointment, so I asked her to wait till a slot opened up. My clients know how busy my days are; if I'm not attending to them in person at the clinic, I'm on the phone counselling them. She waited from 12.30 p.m. to 2 p.m. And when I had a spot of free time, I sat down with her.

Richa, a twenty-nine-year-old weighing at 102.5 kilos, was a successful media personality. I sensed her desperation before she even spoke.

'Nishi,' she said to me, 'you are my only hope. Because I'm convinced I'm never going to lose this weight that I put on.'

I asked her to tell me her history. And after an hour of talking, I was stunned. Richa had done every diet possible in the world! From papaya diets to wine diets to even bizarre things like an idli diet—Richa had tried it all. And failed. Every time she tried something new she would lose a few kilos and promptly put them back on if she faltered even a little. And the amount she would lose was so minuscule that she was always left feeling disheartened.

She had a huge problem—binge eating. And her particular demon was chocolates. Her weakness was that she was an inconsistent dieter, one who fell prey to the joys of eating in a heartbeat.

I knew she was going to be a tough cookie. But I took her on. Within a month of joining my programme, she lost 10 to 12 kilos. Most of it was water weight as she had a huge water retention problem. But this quickly boosted her morale, as results always do, and she persevered even harder. The weight lost kept her motivated.

But things took a turn when she had to leave the programme. Her kids and work pulled her back to the world of easy gratification. I was sad to let her go but ces't la vie, right?

One day, Richa came back. She had put on some more weight and this time she said that she was going the whole hog. Cut to six months later, she left me at 66 kilos, feeling lighter, happier and looking more energetic and radiant. Today, she leads a fulfilling life, because of the tremendous change in her weight. And I am happy that I had a small part to play in it.

If you are 10 to 20 kilos over your ideal weight, I urge you not to despair. In all my years as a dietician and trainer, I've seen some of the most drastic of cases lose weight and reach their ideal weight.

If Richa can do it, so can you!

The best good news is that no matter what your weight loss goal is, even a modest weight loss, such as 5 kilos will better your blood sugar, blood pressure and blood cholesterol levels. You're doing this for the long haul. Try to think of it as an investment in your health.

For example, if you currently weigh 90 kilos and you bring your weight down even to 80 kilos, it can decrease the risk factor for chronic diseases related to obesity. You may still be overweight but even such a modest and slim drop results in nothing but benefits to your body. Imagine, losing 20 kilos then? Think how beneficial it will be for you in the long run?

So even if the overall goal seems large, see it as a journey rather than just a final destination. You'll learn new eating and physical activity habits that will help you live a healthier lifestyle. These habits may help you maintain your weight loss over time.

In addition to improving your health, maintaining a weight loss diet is likely to improve your life in other ways. Not only will your overall physical health improve, here are some other positive factors that you'll enjoy:

The Other Gains of Weight Loss

- Increase in overall energy levels
- Greater physical mobility
- Increase in confidence
- Skin and hair become better—more glow, more lush
- Even small changes like less flatulence in the mornings
- No bloatedness
- Face will be less puffy
- Spring in your step
- Better mood

Drink lots of water. You have to drink at least eight glasses of water each day. If you feel you can't drink so much water, try jasmine or chamomile tea and eat foods with a high water content such as cucumbers. Keep in mind that caffeine and chai are dehydrating.

MEAL PLAN 1

Time	Food
On rising 6.30 a.m.	Fresh coriander and tulsi leaves (2–4) soaked overnight; strain the leaves and drink the water + 1 tsp aloe vera juice diluted in a glass of water + Warm water with flax seeds powder and ¼ tsp of watermelon, sunflower and pumpkin seeds
7. 30 a.m.	Green/regular tea (optional)
Breakfast between 8 and 8.30 a.m.	Skimmed milk (100 ml) + Muesli (sugar-free and without any dried fruit)
10 a.m.	1–2 strawberries
11–11.30 a.m.	Mixed salad
Lunch between 12–1 p.m.	Oat flour + oat bran stuffed roti (methi/gobi/palak/mixed vegetables) + Oil-free vegetables (no corn and potato)
2 p.m.	¼ piece of mausambi
3–3.30 p.m.	Tea/coffee (with 2 tsp of skimmed milk) + 2 cream crackers (Brittania)
5 p.m.	Mixed green salad
6 p.m.	1 oats idli + Fresh tomato rasam with beans and drumsticks

MEAL PLAN 2

Time	Food
On rising 7–7.30 a.m.	Fresh coriander and tulsi leaves (2–4) soaked overnight; strain the leaves and drink the water + 1 tsp aloe vera juice diluted in a glass water + ¼ tsp mixed seeds + 1 tsp flax seeds powder
8 a.m.	100 ml soy milk (plain, unflavoured) + 1 Weetabix
9.30 a.m.	¼ piece of green apple
11 a.m.	Mixed green salad (without potato, sprouts, corn or tofu) (no oil-based dressings)
12.30 p.m.	Quinoa veg. pulao (200 gms of quinoa grain) + Vegetables + Green chutney
2 p.m.	¼ piece of mausambi
3 p.m.	Green tea/regular tea/coffee (2 tsp skimmed milk, no sugar) + 2 Marie Lite biscuits
4.30 p.m.	¼ piece of orange
5.30–6 p.m.	1 slice multigrain bread + 2 egg whites with vegetables (scrambled)

Coming Up Next

The wait is over! The next chapter is a tiny recipe book filled with nutritious and super healthy oil-free recipes to get you that glowing skin that you've always desired.

DETOX PLANS

Two weeks after you've transitioned into the diet is the ideal time for a detox. Detoxification is a time-tested dietary plan that helps flush toxins from your body and allows your digestive system much needed rest. Today, we generally eat more than the natural calorie requirements, and in doing so we burden our vital organs, overloading the liver and gut. Just like you look forward to the weekend after five hectic and gruelling workdays, your body, too, needs some rest. Think of a detox as a much needed weekend for your body.

Detoxing has acquired a bad reputation over the years as people think it's akin to starvation. The idea behind the detox plans is to cleanse the system of impurities and give it foods and juices that take minimum effort to digest and process. I always make sure my clients do half a day of detox after two weeks of the diet so that they, too, can get its benefits. A detox has less to do with weight loss and is for the rejuvenation of the body. Complement your detox with lots of water—this will intensify the process of flushing out toxins and also keep you hydrated through the day. A note of caution: do not attempt to do too many detoxes in a week; it should be done maximum once or twice a month. Also, if you suffer from low blood pressure, or any other illness, check with your doctor if the detox plan is right for you.

The benefits of detoxing are so huge that it's become a million-dollar industry. Its presence is also trickling into India with new companies offering pre-made cold pressed natural raw juices for different times of the day. You can buy these packages for a day or a whole week. The benefits of detoxing are plenty. From glowing skin, to increased alertness and vitality, anyone who has done a detox will rave about its many perks.

I've outlined two detox plans for you to choose from. Since now you are aware of what foods you should be eating and which ones to avoid during the diet, you can adapt the fruits to your taste. The simplest way to remember which fruits you should be eating is: if it's too sweet, then it's not the fruit for you at the moment. Mangoes, litchis, custard apple and the like are a no no.

DETOX PLAN 1

Time	Food
6 a.m.	30 ml fresh wheat grass juice diluted in a glass of water
	+
	1 tsp of barley soaked in a glass of water overnight
	+
	1 tsp of aloe vera juice diluted in a glass of water
	+
	¼ tsp of pumpkin, melon, watermelon seeds

The Bridal Diet

Time	Food
8 a.m.	Fresh coconut water
8.30 a.m.	1 green apple
9.30 a.m.	¼ orange
11 a.m.	Fresh coconut water
12.30 p.m.	1 banana
2 p.m.	¼ orange
3.30 p.m.	Juice of 2 mausambis + 3 almonds
5 p.m.	½ pear
6. 30 p.m.	½ green apple

DETOX PLAN 2

Time	Food
7–7.30 am	1 tsp of aloe vera juice diluted in a glass of water + 30 ml fresh wheat grass juice diluted in a glass of water + Fresh coconut water
8.30 a.m.	Juice of celery, carrot, green apple, cucumber and alpha alpha grass
10 a.m.	Sweet lime juice
1 p.m.	Cucumber juice
3 p.m.	Bottle gourd (ghiya) juice
4.30 p.m.	Cucumber juice
6 p.m.	Orange + apple juice

FOLLOW-UP DIET AFTER DETOX

Time	Food
6 a.m.	1 tsp of aloe vera juice diluted in a glass of water + Chia seeds, flax seeds powder, pumpkin seeds, melon seeds, sunflower seeds (1 tsp each) + ½ lemon in warm water + 3 almonds (soaked overnight)
8 a.m.	Fresh coconut water + 1 oat khakra
10 a.m.	½ orange
11–11.30 a.m.	Raw mixed green salad
12 p.m.	Oats pulao (khichdi) (1 tbsp oats) + 1 katori dahi
1.30 p.m.	Fresh coconut water + 2 figs
4 p.m.	½ orange
5 p.m.	½ orange

9

Oil-free Recipes for a Beautiful Bride

'Let food be thy medicine and medicine be thy food'—
Hippocrates

After I published my first book *Lose a Kilo a Week,* I was inundated with mails, phone calls and visits to my clinic by people who loved the idea of oil-free cooking. Most of them were just surprised that they could make the same foods they were eating daily but in a healthier way. They called saying they loved the recipes and wanted more! It thrilled me to see people adapting their way of eating with a little bit of guidance. After all, everyone can be fit and healthy if only they knew how to!

Indian food, yum as it is, can also go overboard on the spices and oil. Most of our vegetables are cooked till they have zero nutritional value left. So what then are we essentially eating, if you cook your vegetables for an hour on full heat? Dead stuff basically. My twist on our daily recipes is healthy, nutritious, and beyond doubt, still has the yum factor. In this chapter, I'm giving you a whole host of recipes to choose from and adapt into your daily cooking. I've taken care to select ingredients that are easily available at your local market. There's nothing here that your local sabziwallah can't cough up. Brides and brides-to-be, especially, can benefit a lot from these super healthy, nutritious and delicious recipes. So go ahead and give them a try. I guarantee you will be asking for more.

SOUPS

1. Warm Winter Tomato and Basil Soup
Serves: 4
Ingredients

250 gm tomatoes
2 small onions
3 cloves of garlic
1 bay leaf
A handful of fresh basil leaves
1 cup of skimmed milk
A pinch of crushed black pepper
Salt to taste

How to
- Bung the tomatoes, onions, garlic cloves, bay leaf and salt in a pressure cooker, and cook till the tomatoes are tender.
- Once they are cooked, allow it cool. Remove the bay leaf and put the mixture into a blender. Blend till it is of a smooth consistency.

- Strain out the tomato seeds.
- Put the mixture into a saucepan, add the basil, a cup of milk and the black pepper.
- Check for salt and serve hot.

2. Hearty Green Pea Soup
Serves: 4
Ingredients

½ kg green peas

A few twigs of rosemary

1 tbsp garlic paste

A handful of fresh basil leaves

A pinch of crushed black pepper

Salt to taste

How to
- First we'll make a flavourful stock. The secret behind any yummy soup or curry is its stock.
- Boil half of the peas, with the rosemary, garlic paste, basil and salt in a pressure cooker till it is tender.
- Once it's done, allow it to cool.
- Put the mixture into a blender, and blend till it is of a smooth consistency.
- Strain out the chunky bits using a fine sieve.
- Now boil the remaining peas. Once they are done, blend them till they are of a smooth consistency.
- Add the stock to the blended peas and stir it well.

- Garnish with crushed black pepper and check for salt.
- Serve hot.

3. Refreshing Lemon and Coriander Soup
Serves: 4
Ingredients

A bunch of celery

2 cups vegetable stock

1 inch Thai ginger

½ tsp garlic

Green chillies according to taste

½ tsp coriander seeds

1 bunch of fresh coriander

100 gm beans

150 gm carrots

1 small floret of broccoli

Quarter piece of bell peppers

1 tbsp soya sauce

2 tsp lemon juice

1tbsp vinegar

½ tsp lemongrass

Salt to taste

100 gm carrots

150 asparagus

150 gm broccoli

A few cabbage leaves

A lemon rind

How to

- Boil the celery in 2 cups of water with ginger, garlic, green chillies, coriander seeds, fresh coriander and vegetable stock.
- Let this cook for 30 minutes on low heat with the lid on.
- Once this is done, strain the water out and reserve for later.
- Cut the vegetables into thin slivers.
- Add the freshly cut vegetables, a splash of soya sauce, lemon juice, vinegar, green chillies, lemon grass and lemon rind to the stock. Cook it a little bit.
- Add cut chillies and serve hot.

4. Robust Mushroom Soup

Serves: 4

Ingredients

1 packet button mushroom

1 bay leaf

1½ cups water

½ tsp garlic

Green chillies according to taste

Salt to taste

½ cup skimmed milk

A few slices of wholegrain bread

A pinch of crushed black pepper

How to

- Clean and quarter the mushrooms.

- Next, add 1 ½ cups of water into the pressure cooker, and add the mushrooms (leave some aside), bay leaf, garlic and green chillies.
- Turn it off after one whistle and allow it to cool.
- Blend it into a thick puree in the blender and add the milk.
- Boil the remaining mushrooms till tender and add them to the soup.
- Add pepper and a few baked croutons and serve hot.

To make the croutons:
- Take a few slices of bread and cut them into small squares.
- Slather a bit of garlic paste and pepper on them.
- Bake it in the oven for 15 to 20 minutes or till they are crisp.

5. Mixed Vegetable Soup
Serves: 4
Ingredients

250 gm carrots

200 gm spinach

200 gm onions

100 gm beans

100 gm cabbage

1 tbsp ginger–garlic paste

1 stick cinnamon

1–2 cloves

A pinch of nutmeg

Green chillies according to taste

500 ml skimmed milk
A bunch of fresh coriander
Salt to taste
A pinch of garam masala

How to

- Bung in all the vegetables, ginger–garlic paste and the spices except the garam masala in a pressure cooker and cook till they are done.
- Allow it to cool, then blend it into a thick puree in the blender.
- Add 500 ml of milk to this. The milk will give it a nice creamy thickness.
- Let this mixture boil on low heat for 45 minutes.
- Add the garam masala for garnish.
- Check for salt. Garnish with coriander and serve hot.

6. Spinach and Mushroom Soup

Serves: 4

Ingredients

200 gm spinach
500 ml of vegetable stock
1 packet of button mushrooms
250 gm onions
Garlic paste (roasted)
Green chillies according to taste
1 bay leaf

½ litre skimmed milk

A pinch of oregano

Some basil leaves

A pinch of crushed black pepper

Baked croutons

Salt to taste

How to

- Wash the spinach and mushrooms properly and then chop them roughly.
- Put the vegetable stock in a pressure cooker and add the vegetables, garlic paste, green chillies, salt and bay leaf.
- Once they are cooked, remove the bay leaf and allow to cool.
- Blend this into a thick puree in the blender.
- Add the milk and cook on low heat for 30 minutes.
- Garnish with oregano, basil and black pepper.
- Serve hot with baked croutons (For crouton recipe, see p 88).

7. Pumpkin Soup

Serves: 4

Ingredients

500 gm pumpkin

250 gm onions

1 tsp garlic (roasted)

Green chillies according to taste

1 bay leaf

½ litre skimmed milk

Pinch of oregano

Some basil leaves

A pinch of crushed black pepper

Baked croutons

Salt to taste

How to

- Cut the pumpkin into cubes and put it in a pressure cooker, along with the onions, roasted garlic, bay leaf, green chillies and salt. Cook it till it's done.
- Once they are cooked, remove the bay leaf and allow to cool.
- Blend into a thick puree in a blender.
- Add the milk and cook on low heat for 30 minutes.
- Garnish with oregano, basil and black pepper.
- Serve hot with baked croutons (For crouton recipe, see p 88).

8. Nourishing Broccoli and Spinach Soup

Serves: 4

Ingredients

250 gm broccoli

250 gm spinach

150 gm spring onions

1 tsp garlic and ginger paste

Nishi Grover

1 bay leaf
1 stick cinnamon
1–2 cloves
1 big cardamom
Green chillies according to taste
½ tsp jeera
150 ml skimmed milk
A pinch of crushed black pepper
Baked croutons
Salt to taste

How to
- Wash and clean the vegetables thoroughly and then cut them.
- Boil the vegetables in 3 cups of water and add the ginger and garlic paste, bay leaf, cinnamon, cloves and big cardamom.
- Add the salt and a bit of the green chillies.
- Once they are cooked, remove the bay leaf and other spices and allow it to cool.
- Blend into a thick puree in the blender.
- Add the jeera and the milk. Let it boil for a while so that it thickens.
- Check for salt.
- Add the pepper and serve hot with the baked croutons (For crouton recipe, see p 88).

9. High Protein Egg Drop and Clear Chicken and Veg Soup

Serves: 4

Ingredients

A) For the stock:

½ kg chicken bones

1 tsp lemon grass

1 tsp garlic paste

6–8 kafir leaves

1 inch Thai ginger

A dash of lemon rind

5 stalks celery

1 tsp coriander seeds

1 bunch fresh coriander stem

Salt to taste

B) For the soup

A few leaves of cabbage

100 gm carrots

150 gm asparagus

150 gm broccoli

200 gm shredded chicken breast

Green chillies according to taste

1 tbsp lemon grass

1 tbsp light soya sauce

A bunch of coriander leaves

A dash of lemon rind

A pinch of crushed black pepper
2 egg whites
Juice of 1 lemon
Salt to taste

How to
- Boil all the ingredients of A in a pan of water and remove the scum as and when it rises to the surface. Allow this to cook for at least an hour, till the water reduces.
- When this is done, sieve the stock, throwing away the bones, leaves and spices, and keep the stock on boil.
- In the meantime, cut all the vegetables into slivers and then add it to the stock and cook for a bit.
- Boil the chicken breast till it's cooked. Allow it to cool and then shred it.
- Add salt and green chillies, fresh coriander leaves, lemon grass, a splash of light soya sauce, some grated lemon rind and black pepper.
- Add the shredded chicken and the egg whites to the stock and stir vigorously.
- Add the lemon juice.
- Serve hot.

10. Curd and Besan Shorba
Serves: 4
Ingredients

½ litre curd
500 ml water

The Bridal Diet

1 tbsp besan
Green chillies (deseeded) according to taste
A bunch of fresh coriander
Salt to taste

Spices

A pinch of hing
½ tsp black mustard seeds
1 inch ginger
A few curry leaves
½ tsp methi dana

How to
- Add water to the curd and beat it well. There should be no lumps in it.
- Sieve the besan and add it to the curd.
- In a pan, roast all the spices for a few minutes, and add it to the curd and besan mixture.
- Now add the chillies in this.
- Cook the curd and besan mixture on low heat for 45 minutes covered. Stir it from time to time.
- Check for salt. Garnish with coriander and serve hot.

Nishi Grover

SALADS

1. Lime and Mint Salad
Serves: 4
Ingredients

Curd made with ½ litre skimmed milk

1 tsp lemongrass

1 tsp grated ginger juice

A dash of grated lemon rind

1 tbsp orange juice

A pinch of crushed black pepper

Salt to taste

1 tsp Splenda (sugar substitute)

A bunch of fresh coriander

A few mint leaves

Baked croutons

How to

- Hang the curd in a thin muslin cloth until it thickens.
- Mix all the other ingredients (except coriander and mint) together well. Then add to the curd.
- Garnish with coriander, mint and baked croutons (For crouton recipe, see p 88).
- Serve chilled.

2. Pizza Salad

Serves: 4

Ingredients

A) For the base:

2 tbsp oat bran flour

A pinch of jeera

A pinch of ajwain

½ tsp garlic paste

Salt to taste

B) For the sauce:

100 gm tomato pulp

250 gm tomato puree (cooked)

A pinch of crushed black pepper

1 tsp garlic paste

Tabasco according to taste

A pinch of Splenda

Chilli flakes according to taste

Pizza herbs such as rosemary, thyme and basil

Green chillies according to taste

Salt to taste

How to

- Mix all the ingredients of A well and make it into a pliable dough.
- Roll out small thin rotis and bake them in the oven for 15 minutes or till done.

97

- Then, in a pan, add the tomato pulp and puree and mix well.
- Add all the other ingredients of B (except Tabasco, coriander and pizza herbs) and cook for 2 minutes on low heat.
- In the end, add the Tabasco and coriander.
- Garnish with pizza herbs.
- Serve hot.

3. Papri Chaat Salad

Serves: 4

Ingredients

A) For the papri:

2 tbsp oat flour

2 tbsp rice flour

Salt to taste

A pinch of ajwain

B) For the green chutney:

A bunch of fresh mint leaves

6 stems of coriander

2 green chillies or as per taste

½ small onion

2 tbsp dahi

Lemon juice or 1 whole anardana

How to

Combine all the ingredients for B) and grind to a smooth paste in a blender using very little water.

C) For the tamarind chutney:

1 tbsp tamarind (soak it in hot water for a while and then
extract the pulp and strain it)
1 ½ tbsp Splenda
A pinch of garam masala
Salt and red chilli powder to taste
Bhuna jeera to taste

How to

Take all the ingredients and blend it well in a blender.

D) For the vegetable paste:

100 gm petha/kaddu (boiled and mashed)
½ small onion
1 tbsp moong daal
Coriander leaves
Green chillies according to taste

How to

Mix the first three ingredients together and add the coriander
and green chillies and salt.

E) The curd:

Curd made out of ½ litre skimmed milk
Salt to taste
Jeera powder and ajwain to taste

How to:

Set the curd the night before. Beat it well and add the jeera,
ajwain powder and salt.

F) Others:

Cucumber

Tomato

Lettuce

Carrot

Beetroot

Mint

Coriander

As much as you require

How to

- Mix the ingredients of A and make a tight dough with some water.
- Roll out a big roti, and using a knife or a cutter, cut out small papris. Prick them with a knife.
- Bake them in the oven at 180 degrees for 10 to 15 minutes or till they are done.
- Apply the paste mixture on the papris, and add the finely chopped vegetables.
- Arrange the papris on a plate and add all three chutneys on each papri.
- Garnish with fresh mint and coriander.
- Serve chilled.

4. Lebanese Babaganoush Salad

Serves: 4

Ingredients

1 medium-sized brinjal (roasted, skinned and pulped)

1 litre hung curd (made from skimmed milk)

The Bridal Diet

Juice of 1 lemon
A dash of grated lemon rind
A pinch of crushed black pepper
A pinch of white pepper
2 tsp roasted white sesame seeds
½ tsp garlic paste (roasted)
1 tbsp boiled chickpea puree
Salt to taste
A bunch of coriander

How to

- Make tiny pricks all over the skin of the brinjal and roast it over the gas for a while. Ensure that the brinjal is roasted completely from the inside.
- Remove the burnt skin and mash the pulp completely.
- In a bowl, mix the curd, brinjal pulp, chickpea puree, black and white pepper, garlic, lemon juice and rind and salt. Mix this well.
- Sprinkle sesame seeds and coriander over the mixture.
- Serve immediately.
- This can also be served as a dip with sticks of cucumber and carrots.

5. Lebanese Green Pea Salad

Serves: 4

Ingredients

Curd made from 500 ml of skimmed milk
250 gm green peas

1 red pepper (roast it and remove the dead skin)
1 tsp roasted garlic
½ tsp black pepper
½ tsp white pepper
A pinch of chilli flakes
A dash of grated lemon rind
1 small ball of iceberg lettuce
1 cucumber (grated)
1 tbsp white sesame paste
Salt to taste
Baked croutons

How to
- Hang the curd in a muslin cloth to remove any excess liquid. Once it thickens, your curd is ready.
- Boil the peas and puree them in a blender into a thick paste.
- Add the curd to the peas.
- Roast the red pepper and remove the charred skin and seeds. Add the pepper pulp to the curd and peas mixture.
- Now add the roasted garlic, black pepper, white pepper, salt, chilli flakes and lemon rind.
- Check for salt.
- Add the iceberg lettuce, grated cucumber, white sesame paste.
- Add the baked croutons (For crouton recipe, see p 88) and serve chilled.

6. Crunchy Thai Salad

Serves: 4

Ingredients

250 gm tomato puree

1 tbsp light soya sauce

1 inch Thai ginger

5–6 kafir leaves

1 tbsp vinegar

1 tbsp Thai red curry paste

10–20 peanuts (roasted)

10–12 almonds

½ packet noodles

A pinch of crushed black pepper

1 tsp white sesame seeds (roasted)

Salt to taste

How to

- Puree the tomatoes and strain it well to remove the skin and seeds. Ensure that it is of a smooth consistency.
- Add the soya sauce, Thai ginger, kafir leaves, vinegar, Thai red curry paste (after straining the oil out).
- Add the peanuts, crushed black pepper, sesame seeds and salt.
- Cut the almonds into thin slivers and roast them along with the noodles. Then bake them in the oven till it turns brown.
- Blend the peanuts and sesame seeds. This is the dressing. Add this to the salad.
- Top the salad with the noodles and almond crunch and serve chilled.

7. Summery Golguppa Salad

Serves: 4

Ingredients

A) For the dough

½ cup oat flour

Enough milk to make the dough

A pinch ajwain

Salt to taste

B) For the paste

½ cup moong daal (boiled)

2 small onions

Salt to taste

A small bunch of fresh coriander

1 tsp lemon juice

Green chillies according to taste

C) For the coriander and mint chutney

A bunch of fresh coriander

A bunch of fresh mint

1 tsp lemon juice

Salt to taste

Chillies according to taste

1 whole pomegranate (deseeded)

500 ml curd

D) For the tamarind chutney

1 tbsp of tamarind paste

3 tsp Splenda

Salt to taste

A pinch of garam masala

½ tsp jeera powder

E) For the salad

2 tomatoes

250 gm petha (boiled)

1 cucumber

F) For the jal jeera water

Water

1 tsp mint and coriander paste

1 inch ginger

Salt to taste

Green chillies according to taste

1 tsp bhuna jeera

A few fresh mint leaves

A bunch of fresh coriander

How to

- Take all the ingredients of A and make a tight dough.
- Cut out small circular discs using a cutter.
- Take a lemon and wrap a dough disc around it so that it is fully enveloped. Make as many as you want.
- Bake the balls till they turn brown. Once done, gently remove the lemons.
- Take all the ingredients of B, mix well and keep aside.

- Combine all the ingredients of F, mix well and keep aside.
- Take all the ingredients of C and blend well in a blender. Make sure the consistency is thin enough to spread.
- Take all the ingredients of D and blend well in a blender.
- Now once you've prepared all your chutneys and pastes, take the golguppa balls and fill them with the moong daal mixture.
- Add the salad on top, then drizzle both the chutneys, and lastly, the jal jeera.
- Serve chilled.

8. Spicy Mexican Salad
Serves: 4

Ingredients

A) For the nachos

You can buy readymade nachos from the store or make your own low-calorie wheat nachos at home.

B) For the salsa

250 gm tomatoes

Juice of 1 lemon

A bunch of coriander

Black pepper to taste

White pepper to taste

Pulp of 1 avocado

½ tsp sweetener

A couple drops of Tabasco sauce
5–7 salad sticks
Salt to taste

How to

- To make the nachos, first make a few rotis. Then, cut small circles out of them using a cutter.
- Bake them in a chapati maker after adding jeera and ajwain in the roti till they are done.
- Take the tomatoes and roast them in the oven till they are done.
- Remove from oven and peel off the skins of the tomatoes and then pulp them.
- Add all the other ingredients to the pulp.
- Serve with salad sticks and the baked nachos.

9. Italian Balsamic Vinegar Salad

Serves: 4

Ingredients

A) For the dressing

3 tbsp balsamic vinegar
1 tsp orange peel (without the pits)
A dash of grated lemon rind
French mustard according to taste
A pinch of crushed black pepper
A pinch of white pepper
½ tsp mustard powder
Salt to taste

B) For the salad

Cut as much as you need of these vegetables

Romaine lettuce

Iceberg lettuce

Baby spinach

Olives

Bell peppers

Cucumber

Blanched broccoli

Jalapeno

Cherry tomatoes

Gherkins

How to

- Heat the balsamic vinegar on low heat for 10 minutes to thicken it.
- Take the orange peel and cut it into thin slivers. Then bake it in the oven till its crisp.
- Combine all the ingredients of A to make the dressing.
- Cut all the vegetables into small cubes and shred the leafy ones to make the salad.
- Add the dressing to the salad.
- Serve chilled.

10. Cool Mediterranean Salad

Serves: 4

Ingredients

A) For the dressing

500 ml of curd made out of skimmed milk

The Bridal Diet

1 tbsp chickpea puree
100 gm fresh methi pulp
1 tsp mustard paste
A pinch of mustard powder

B)   1 tsp ginger garlic paste
Sweetener according to taste
Green chillies (deseeded and pureed) according to taste
Salt to taste

C) For the salad

Cut as much as you need of these vegetables

Carrots

Lettuce

Olives

Bell peppers

Cucumber

Tomatoes

½ tsp roasted sunflower seeds

½ tsp roasted pumpkin seeds

How to

- Hang the curd in a muslin cloth till all the excess water is drained and the curd is thick.
- Add all the ingredients of A to the curd and mix well.
- Now add the ginger garlic paste, sweetener, green chillies, and salt. Your dressing is now ready.

- Cut the vegetables into small bits to make the salad.
- Now, add the dressing to freshly cut vegetables.
- Sprinkle some roasted sunflower and pumpkin seeds over the salad and serve chilled.

11. Korean Kimchi Salad

Serves: 4

Ingredients

A) For the dressing

250 gm tomato puree (fresh)

1 tbsp light soya sauce

1 tbsp vinegar

½ tsp roasted coriander seeds

1 stick cinnamon

½ tsp ginger garlic paste

½ tsp each black and white sesame seeds (roasted)

½ packet noodles (roasted)

½ tsp honey

Salt to taste

B) For the salad

Cut as much as you need of these vegetables

Cabbage

Carrots

Lettuce

French beans

1 tbsp roasted peanuts

1 tbsp roasted cashew nuts

How to

- Puree the tomatoes in a blender and keep aside.
- Now roast all the dry spices on a pan and then grind them into a fine powder.
- Add the spices to the tomato puree and mix well to make a fine dressing.
- Cut the vegetables into small bits to make the salad.
- Now, add the dressing to freshly cut vegetables.
- Roast the noodles and top it off on the salad for an extra crunch.
- Sprinkle the peanuts and cashew nuts at the end and serve.

MAINS

1. Smacky South Indian Rasam

Serves: 4

Ingredients

500 gm tomatoes

A pinch of hing

1 tbsp black mustard seeds

1 tbsp curry patta

1 tsp ginger–garlic paste

1 tsp tamarind (soaked and pulped)

1 tsp rasam powder

1 tsp chutney powder

1 tsp sambhar powder

Salt to taste

How to

- Boil the tomatoes until they are soft. Then puree the tomatoes and strain out the skin and seeds through a fine sieve.
- In a pan, roast hing, mustard seeds, curry patta and the ginger-garlic paste.
- Pour in the tomato puree and tamarind into the seasoning.
- Cook for 30 to 45 minutes on low heat.
- Once this is done, add the chutney, rasam and sambhar powders.
- Garnish with curry patta and a dash of mustard seeds.
- Serve hot.

2. Punjabi Dahi ki Kadhi

Serves: 4

Ingredients

1 litre curd made out of skimmed milk

2 cups water

1 tbsp roasted besan

A pinch of hing

1 inch of chopped ginger

A pinch of haldi

½ tsp methi seeds

½ tsp black mustard seeds (dry roasted)

A bit of curry patta

Green chillies to taste

Salt to taste

For the pakoras

1 to 3 tbsp besan
500 gm chopped onions
½ tsp anardana
Green chillies to taste
Coriander to garnish
A bit of methi

How to

- Set the curd the night before and allow it to turn sour.
- Before cooking, beat the curd well and add 1 ½ cups of besan.
- Mix it in a blender.
- Pour out this mixture in a pan and put it on medium flame.
- Add 2 cups of water.
- Then add hing, ginger, haldi, methi seeds, mustard seeds and curry patta.
- Cook for one hour till it thickens.
- In the meantime, make the pakoras. Make a thick batter with all the ingredients and then make small balls out of it.
- Roast them in the oven till they turn brown.
- Once the kadhi is almost done, add the pakoras into the kadhi.
- Serve hot with boiled rice.

3. Dahi Vada

Serves: 4

Ingredients

1 litre curd made out of skimmed milk
½ cup green moong daal

250 gm onions
Coriander to garnish
Green chillies according to taste
½ tsp cooking soda
Salt to taste

How to

- Soak the moong daal for a few hours till it is soft.
- Grind the daal and stir it vigorously with a wooden spoon and some cooking soda. Keep this vada mixture aside for 45 minutes.
- In the meantime, chop the onions and mix it in the moong daal mixture. Stir for a few minutes.
- Add salt, fresh coriander and green chillies.
- Pre-heat the oven at 200 degrees Celsius and place the vada mixture on the tray, making a hole in the centre. Turn it after a few minutes.
- Now beat the curd till it is of a smooth consistency and add the vadas in the curd.
- Serve chilled with a crunch of baked boondi.

4. Matar Paneer Gravy

Serves: 4

Ingredients

1 litre skimmed milk for the paneer
250 gm tomatoes
250 gm chopped onions
1 bay leaf
1 stick of cinnamon

2 to 3 cardamoms (big and small)
½ tsp jeera
1 Kashmiri mirch
500 gm peas
½ tsp kasoori methi
Coriander to garnish
Salt to taste

How to

- Make low-fat paneer with 1 litre milk. Flatten it and cut it into cubes.
- Blanch the tomatoes till they are soft and puree them in a blender. Sieve the puree properly, discarding the skin and seeds. Ensure that it's not lumpy.
- Sauté the onions and puree it separately.
- In a non-stick pan, cook the onions and tomatoes until they turn deep reddish brown.
- In a clean pan, put a bay leaf, cinnamon, cardamom (big and small), jeera, Kashmiri mirch, and add the tomato puree. Cover the pan and let this cook for 45 minutes. Add a bit of water while cooking.
- Add peas while cooking the tomato and onion mixture.
- Now add the paneer to the gravy.
- Roast each piece of paneer in a non-stick pan lightly.
- Add the gravy and allow it cook together for a bit.
- Check for salt and add kasoori methi.
- Garnish with coriander before serving.

5. Shahi Paneer
Serves: 4
Ingredients

500 gm tomatoes

250 gm onions

½ tsp ginger–garlic paste

200 gm paneer or tofu

½ tsp coconut powder

10 to 12 pureed cashew nuts

1 litre skimmed milk to make the paneer

500 ml skimmed milk

Coriander to garnish

A few sesame seeds

Salt to taste

How to
- First make low-fat paneer with 1 litre milk. Flatten it and cut it into cubes.
- Boil the tomatoes till they are soft and puree them in a blender. Sieve the puree to remove lumps.
- Chop the onions roughly and sauté it with ginger, garlic, pureed cashew nuts and salt.
- Puree the onions and add to the tomato puree.
- To make the gravy creamy, puree 200 gm of paneer or tofu, and add it to the tomatoes.
- To this, add the coconut powder and sesame seeds and cook for 2 hours on low heat to thicken it.
- Now add the paneer cubes to the gravy.

- When the gravy cools, add 500 ml of cold skimmed milk and stir it.
- Garnish with coriander and serve hot.

6. Mixed Vegetable Keema Kebab

Serves: 4

Ingredients

½ cup channa daal

250 gm carrots

250 gm pumpkin

250 gm spinach

2 large cardamom pods

1–2 cloves

1–2 cinnamon

A pinch of star anise

½ tsp jeera (roasted)

¼ tsp coriander powder

A pinch of kasoori methi

Salt to taste

How to

- Boil the daal in a pan till it is cooked.
- Chop all the vegetables finely and bung them into the pressure cooker. Cook till they are soft.
- Add the boiled and mashed daal into the pressure cooker. Make sure that there is no extra water in this.

117

- Roast the cardamom pods, cloves, cinnamon, star anise, jeera, coriander powder and kasoori methi.
- Now grind the roasted spices and add them to the vegetables and daal.
- Make small round balls of the mixture and roast them on a non-stick pan. Don't move the kebabs around too much or they'll break. Make sure they're cooked properly then flip them over.
- Serve hot with pudina chutney.

7. South Indian Vegetable Kebabs Served on a Crusty Base

Serves: 4

Ingredients
For kebabs:

1 cup kala channa

½ kilo methi

250 gms spring onions

250 gms peas

Roasted cinnamon powder to taste

Parsley to taste

Jeera to taste

Ajwain to taste

Green chillies to taste

Tamarind water

For crusty base:
Bread cut in round shape and baked like a crouton in an oven

100 gms tofu
Salt to taste
A pinch of black pepper

Red chutney:

2–3 dried red chillies
4–5 cloves of garlic
Salt
½ tsp Splenda
2–3 medium tomatoes

How to

- Boil the kala channa and blend it into a paste.
- Cook the methi leaves and finely chopped onions with peas in a non-stick pan till tender.
- Add this mixture to the channa puree and mix well.
- Add roasted cinnamon powder, parsley, jeera, ajwain, green chillies and some tamarind water.
- Now mix well and make them into round balls.
- Bake the balls on a non-stick pan till they turn brown.
- In the meantime, for the red chutney, roast the red chillies and pound them into a rough powder.
- Add tomato puree and the rest of the spices.
- Now put it on low flame and cook it till it becomes thick.
- Keep aside.
- For the tofu paste, blend the tofu with some skimmed milk and make a paste.
- Add some salt and black pepper for taste.

- For the final combination and presentation, place the round cut bread on a plate.
- Apply some tofu paste and red chutney.
- Now place the kebabs on top.
- Again put the red chutney and tofu on the kebabs and serve hot on a plate.

8. Matar Paneer ki Bhurji

Serves: 4

Ingredients

1 kilo peas

Paneer made with 1 litre skimmed milk

250 grams onions

1 kilo tomatoes (½ kilo puree and ½ kilo finely chopped)

½ cup milk

1 tsp coriander powder

½ tsp coriander seeds (roasted)

½ tsp kasoori methi

A handful of fresh coriander

Salt to taste

1–2 Kashmiri mirch

½ tsp roasted freshly ground garam masala

How to

- Cook the finely chopped onions with Kashmiri mirch and coriander seeds.
- Now add the chopped tomatoes and cook on low heat till the masala is made for 45 minutes.

- Add in all the other spices with half a cup of skimmed milk.
- Add boiled peas.
- In the end add the paneer cubes and fresh coriander and serve hot.

9. Makhani Kali Daal

Serves: 4

Ingredients

½ cup kali daal (soaked overnight)

750 gms tomato puree

3 medium onions

1 cup skimmed milk

Skimmed milk yoghurt made with 500 ml milk

1 tsp ginger cut in small cubes

½ tsp garlic paste

2–3 cloves

1 bay leaf

1–2 roasted Kashmiri mirch

½ tsp kasoori methi

1–2 black elaichi

2–3 green elaichi

1 stick cinnamon

¼ tsp nutmeg

¼ tsp kasoori mirch

¼ tsp jeera

Salt to taste

How to

- Soak the daal overnight and put it in the pressure cooker with the water it was soaked in.
- Add some extra water with the ginger, garlic, cloves, cardamom, bay leaf and boil it under pressure for two whistles.
- On an open pan, cook the daal with the tomato puree.
- Chop half the onions and puree the other half.
- Add the pureed onion paste.
- Cook on low heat for 4 hours.
- Take out all the spice shells.
- Add the rest of the spices with the salt.
- Now cook for 30–45 minutes.
- Add the milk and hung curd and cook for 25 minutes.
- Now separately sauté the rest of the finely chopped onions.
- Add Kashmiri mirch and jeera to the dal.
- Serve hot with freshly chopped coriander.

10. Steamed or Grilled Fish (served on a bed of steamed vegetables)

Serves: 4

Ingredients

250 grams basa or sole fish

2–3 garlic cloves

1 inch ginger cut in small cubes

Black pepper to taste

White pepper to taste

¼ tsp granulated mustard
½ tsp horseradish sauce
Tabasco sauce (a couple of drops)
Balsamic vinegar (a couple of drops)
Cut as much as you need of these vegetables: broccoli,
squash, asparagus, mushrooms
A few sesame seeds

How to

- Take 250 grams of basa or sole fish.
- Shred the fish and add garlic, ginger, black pepper, white pepper, granulated mustard, horseradish sauce, Tabasco and balsamic vinegar.
- Now bind the fish with your palm and make it like a ball.
- Wrap it in foil and steam it in a steamer or out it in an air frier for 15–20 minutes till it becomes light and crispy.
- Add the same spices to the vegetables (they should be lightly steamed to maintain the crunch): broccoli, squash, asparagus, mushrooms.
- Serve the dish hot with some lightly toasted sesame seeds.

11. Dahi-wala Tandoori Chicken

Serves: 4

Ingredients

4 small chicken breasts
1 cup dahi (hung)
Salt to taste

½ tsp tandoori masala
½ tsp amchoor
Coriander powder
¼ tsp jeera powder
¼ tsp degi mirch powder
¼ tsp garam masala powder
A few coriander leaves
Chaat masala (to taste)
Lemon juice (to taste)

How to

- Marinate the clean chicken breast in dahi and add all the dry masalas.
- Keep aside for 2–3 hours.
- Now pour it out on a non-stick pan on low-medium flame and cook till the water dries up.
- Lower the heat and cover the pan.
- Cook for 25–30 minutes, stirring occasionally as the chicken could break.
- Now add some more beaten hung curd and garnish it with coriander and chaat masala.
- Squeeze some lemon juice if needed.

DESSERTS

1. Chocolate Cake
Ingredients

½ cup flour

½ tsp baking powder

A pinch of baking soda

2 tbsp dark cocoa powder

Hung curd

A dash of vanilla essence

½ cup cooking Splenda

3 eggs

A pinch of salt

How to

- Take ½ cup of flour and sieve it with a pinch of salt, ½ tsp baking powder, a pinch of baking soda and 2 tbsp of dark cocoa powder. Sieve 4 to 5 times to make it light and fluffy.
- Crack the eggs into ½ cup of cooking Splenda and beat them well till the mixture is fluffy.
- Fold this in the flour alternating with hung curd. Use the cut and fold method to mix it.
- Add vanilla essence and put it to bake at 180 degrees Celsius for 40 minutes.
- Take the cake out of the oven and allow it to cool.
- Take the cake out of the baking tin. Slice and serve.

2. Baked Apple Cinnamon Pie
Ingredients

Sugar-free oat biscuits

1 tsp cinnamon powder

6 to 8 raisins

3 walnuts

2 Granny Smith apples

Splenda according to taste

A dash of vanilla essence

How to

- In a baking tin, crumble the biscuits roughly and add cinnamon powder, raisins and walnuts. Bake this for 15 to 20 minutes at 180 degree Celsius till it's done.
- Cut the apples into thin slivers. Sprinkle cinnamon powder, raisins, walnuts and Splenda. Bake it for 15 to 20 minutes at 180 degree Celsius till it's done.
- Layer the baked apples on top of the base of oat biscuits and bake together at 180 degree Celsius till it's done.
- Serve hot with vanilla essence.

3. Chocolate Cake and Cookie Crumble
Ingredients
For the cake:

½ cup flour

½ tsp baking powder

A pinch of baking soda

2 tbsp dark cocoa powder

Hung curd

A dash of vanilla essence

½ cup cooking Splenda

3 eggs

Salt

A few Marie biscuits

Chocolate (melted)

Chocolate sauce

6 to 8 almonds

3 walnuts

How to

- To start off, first make a sugar-free cake (see Chocolate Cake recipe; p 125).
- Cut the cake into four quarters and add melted chocolate and chocolate sauce.
- Now put in the Marie biscuits.
- Cut the almonds and walnuts into slivers.
- Mix the dessert together and top it up with slivered almonds and walnuts.
- Serve chilled.

4. Sugar-free Chocolate Tiramisu
Ingredients

A cake (buy fresh vanilla sponge cake from the market)

500 ml skimmed milk

2 tbsp coffee powder

2 tbsp cocoa powder

2 tbsp hung curd (optional)
A couple drops of vanilla essence
½ cup cooking Splenda
4–5 Marie biscuits
½ to 1 bar chocolate (melted)
½ cup chocolate sauce
5 almonds
3–4 walnuts

How to

Cottage cheese balls

- Take 250 ml of milk and curdle it to form cottage cheese.
- Add coffee powder, vanilla essence and some melted chocolate.
- Add Splenda and make a mixture with a beater.
- Make balls with the mixture and place them on a baking tray and bake for 30 minutes at 180 degree Celsius.
- When they're done, take them out of the oven and allow it to cool.

Chocolate Sauce

- In the meantime, make the sugar-free chocolate sauce. Take 250 ml milk. Take 2 tbsp cocoa powder and dissolve it in 50–60 ml milk. Put the rest of the milk to boil. Before it comes to a boil, pour the cocoa mixture into it, stirring continuously to avoid lumps. Cook till sauce thickens. Add a quarter of melted chocolate to make it more chocolaty. When the mixture cools down, add 2 tbsp Splenda.

Now assemble

- Crush the Marie biscuits.
- Add a bit of butter to it and bake it into a base.
- Take a piece of the sponge cake and soak it in a liquid of coffee powder and water. Keep aside.
- Pour the chocolate sauce to cover the cake.
- Add the cottage cheese balls.
- Again add a bit of melted chocolate.
- Optional: You can add some hung curd for cream.
- Sprinkle some cocoa powder and garnish with nuts.

5. Kesar Elaichi Phirni

Serves: 4

Ingredients

500 ml skimmed milk

2 tbsp soaked rice

2–3 strands kesar soaked in warm milk

Elaichi dana out of 4 green pods

4–5 almonds

4–5 raisins

4 tbsp Splenda

How to

- Take 500 ml of skimmed milk.
- Put it in an open pan and set it to boil.
- In the meantime, grind 2 small tsp of soaked rice and add it to the milk.

Nishi Grover

- Stir continuously and make sure the milk does not stick to the pan.
- Watch the milk thicken gradually.
- To avoid lumps, lower the heat.
- Add 2–3 strands of kesar soaked in warm milk and ground elaichi in the milk and turn off the heat.
- As the mixture cools down, add the Splenda and put the phirni into small earthen cups.
- Garnish with almonds and raisins.
- Serve chilled.

6. Pineapple Pastry
Serves: 4
Ingredients

1 small vanilla sponge cake
4–6 slices of fresh pineapple
4–6 tbsp of fresh pineapple juice
Vanilla and pineapple essence
2½ tbsp custard powder
500 ml skimmed milk

How to
- Get a plain vanilla sponge cake.
- Cut it in squares, almost the size of a pastry.
- Soak the pastry in freshly grated pineapple and juice.
- Keep that soaked cake in the refrigerator.
- In the meantime, take 500 ml skimmed milk.

- Put it to boil for the custard.
- Take 2 ½ tsp of custard powder and make a paste with chilled milk.
- Now add the paste to the boiling milk and stir furiously till it becomes thick like a custard.
- Now wait for it to cool down.
- Take out the soaked cake and cut it horizontally .
- In one half, spoon and spread some custard.
- Top the custard with small pieces of pineapple.
- Put the other half on top and spoon and spread the custard.
- Top it with pineapple pieces and some cherries.
- Keep it in the refrigerator and serve chilled.

Coming Up Next

The next section is all about getting fit. We discuss the most common problem areas that most women face. Be it flabby arms or a tummy that never decreases no matter how many stomach crunches you do—you don't have to be a bride-to-be to understand these annoying problem areas. Do the workouts and watch your body tone and firm up.

Part III

Workout

10

Getting Workout Ready

'A fit, healthy body—that is the best fashion statement'
—**Jess C. Scott**

Most people break into a sweat just thinking of exercise. Working out can often be painful and tiresome. Many of you think of skipping it. Some even start going to the gym but ultimately give up, and then all of what you had lost comes right back! The best way to deal with this is to incorporate a simple exercise routine in your schedule. Remember, the more muscle you have, the more calories you'll burn, even when you're not moving—a good reason to up your strength training. There is no escaping the fact that exercise is a must for getting into shape. It will complement the diet programme you have been on, working faster and more effectively for you to reach your goal.

In fact, for many women D-Day (and the honeymoon) acts as a major reason to get back in shape—something that perhaps they have been putting off for many years. They

135

treat it as the time to finally re-evaluate what they want from themselves and others. If you look at it in another way, you can use your wedding date as a deadline to achieve what you want. You've heard the saying—When the going gets tough, the tough get going. Many studies have shown that most people work better under pressure, or when they are being supervised. The pressures that come with a wedding are immense and looking good is a major part of it. There is no short cut to looking and feeling good. Like everything else, it requires patience, hard work, sincerity and time. So instead of leaving your fitness regime till the end, why don't we work backwards so that you can get fit at your own pace. The more time you have, the more you can accomplish. Without the rush and without the stress. You'll have one less thing to worry about when D-Day arrives. So what are you waiting for, let's get started.

Troublesome Areas

Women are never happy with the way they look. I don't know what it is. Humility? Fishing for compliments? Or just lack of confidence? Compliment any girl or woman on how they look and their immediate reply is not a 'thank you' as it should be but a hurried, 'No. But my legs are sooo fat!' or 'I wish I had a better nose', etc. Every woman has one or two (if not more) things they'd like to change about themselves. From tinniest details such as having thicker eyelashes to bigger dissatisfactions like changing their face structure. We've all seen the lovely actress Renée Zellweger's major facial transformation. That said, there are a few common pesky regions that more or less irk almost all women. These are belly fat, love handles, flabby arms, the bum and thighs. The fitness programme I am going to set for you will first tackle these problems, after which I will set out a general exercise routine that will benefit you no matter what your age is or at what juncture you are at in your life.

Before We Get Started
A few important things to keep in mind and do before you get started on this fitness programme (or any fitness programme for that matter):

1. **A visit to the doctor**: It is imperative that you visit the doctor before you start any workout plan. Especially if you haven't been physically active for a long time. Jumping into a strenuous workout can cause serious damage if your body isn't prepared for it. Also, your blood pressure and vital stats should be normal before starting. Do not ignore this very important step. Only after your doctor has given you the green light should you begin.
2. **Planning your schedule:** You should ideally start your fitness programme four to five months before your wedding day. This will give you enough time to get in shape gradually without resorting to drastic measures. The lead-up to the wedding is so stressful

that you should start training early and then pace up two weeks before the big day. If you don't have that much time, you can even start a fitness programme six weeks before your wedding. You can strengthen and tone some key muscles so that even if you don't lose a significant amount of weight, you will stand taller, you'll have more energy and feel better.

3. **Setting real goals**: A lot of brides make the mistake of wanting to look like someone else altogether in their heads! Believe me when I tell you that I have had many women tell me that on their wedding day they want to look like some actress in some movie. You can't change your basic body type— you are who you are. What you should concentrate on is making your body shape look as flattering as possible and highlighting your best parts. It's a time-tested fashion industry secret. And it works like magic if you add confidence to the mix.

4. **Breaking up your exercise routine**: Stressed about finding an hour for cardio? Studies have shown that breaking your 45-minute cardio session into two or three segments per day is just as effective as doing it all at once.

5. **Keeping hydrated**: I can't stress enough about the importance of being hydrated. When you exercise you lose many essential salts and water. Drink enough

fluids to replenish your lost stock. Water helps the body shed toxins and keeps you from over-snacking during the day.

6. **Warming up and cooling down**: Before any exercise, remember to warm up. It prepares the body for exercising, both physically and mentally. Besides preventing injuries, correct exercise preparation will help you get the best out of your workout. It should be done for a minimum of five minutes. When you are warming up, you are literally warming up your body's temperature. Often a warm up is simply the activity you are about to do but at a slower pace. For example, if you are going to be swimming then you start off with a few slow laps. It should be done in a relaxed state.

The same goes for cooling down. The Shavasana, in yoga, is done after every major asana. This is to ensure that the heartbeat comes back to its normal pace and the muscles relax. Cooling down slows your heartbeat, gets your breathing to its regular rhythm, avoids soreness of muscles, and reduces any risk of lightheadedness. In all my years of teaching aerobics, I have seen many cases where absolutely fit people have injured themselves because they never bothered to cool down and stretch properly after working out. Your cooling down routine can vary. It should involve light aerobic activity and stretching.

7. **Stretching properly**: A good stretch at the start and end of your workout routine will reduce muscle injuries and provide the benefits of an increase in flexibility and joint range of motion, correct exercise posture and relaxed muscles. However, stretching has to be done correctly otherwise this, too, can be harmful for your body. Here are some tips on stretching properly:

    *   Stop if it hurts. Stretching should never hurt. If you have reached a point in your stretch where it hurts, relax to where it feels comfortable and hold the stretch.
    *   Maintain each stretch for 10–30 seconds, or till whenever you can. Holding a stretch for any less won't sufficiently lengthen the muscle. Stretch the muscles gradually and don't force it. Avoid bobbing or bouncing while stretching. This may damage the muscle you are stretching.
    *   Remember to breathe. Breathing is a necessary part of any workout, including stretching.
    *   Practise equality. You should not neglect any side of your body. Make sure you stretch both sides equally, so all of your muscles are evenly ready for action.

8. **Spicing things up**: I love exercise. I got into it when I was a teenager, and tried everything from cycling, yoga, running and aerobics. It stimulates me

like nothing else. I feel that most people don't like to exercise because they consider it a task, an ordeal that needs to be dealt with. That attitude will never work. A routine can quickly become boring. So I suggest you add many elements to your workout. Don't just stick to running or doing yoga. Alternate your regular workout with something new, like joining a dance class or going for a trek! You'll begin to love working out and gradually you will make it a part of your life.

Things You Will Need

- **Yoga mat**: This is a basic mat that you need to do your floor exercises.
- **Dumbbells**: Not more than 3 kilos depending on how much you can carry without it weighing you down.
- **Swiss ball or stability ball**: When it comes to fitness equipment, there's little that works your whole body better. To stay on the ball—literally—you're forced to engage all your muscles, which builds strength and improves stability. It comes pretty cheap too, starting at Rs 400.
- **Bosu ball (optional)**: The Bosu ball is like a Swiss ball but cut in half. It is another piece of equipment that is extremely useful for indoor workouts. However, if you have a Swiss ball then you can skip this.

Nishi Grover

Coming Up Next

The next chapter is aimed at losing those flabby arms—workout plans and cheat tricks that will help you get those arms of your dreams.

142

11

Up in Arms

'The best way to hold a man is in your arms'—**Mae West**

Bat wings or bingo wings, arm jiggle. Call it whatever you want. Flabby arms are a woman's most common complaint. In all my years of working as an aerobics instructor and then a dietician, this is the complaint I hear most often. As much as 90 per cent of my clients, both men and women, ask me how they can lose weight in this region. And sometimes I am asked this even after they've lost around 25 kilos! In all my 30-plus years of working as a nutritionist, this is the most common question I've been asked, 'How do I make my arms thin?' And I understand why. Except for the face and feet, the arms are the most exposed part of your body. Well-toned arms make a huge difference to your overall appearance.

Stubborn and irreversible. Two words commonly associated with arm fat. Flabby arms are a tough problem. Once the fat settles in, it's most likely there to stay if you don't check it. Remember, everything can be fixed, every problem has a solution, but to get to it, you'll need to put in some time and really work it off. Fat in the arms is very difficult to get rid of because of the lack of flexible space for our arms to workout. To add to that, our technologically advanced world doesn't help very much either. Where once we washed our own clothes and dishes, now we have washing machines to do such jobs. At times it seems to me that all we do with our hands these days is type and text. Hain na?

Hollywood celebrity trainer Joe Dowdell in her book *Ultimate You: A 4-Phase Total Body Makeover for Women Who Want Maximum Results*, which is co-authored by Dr Brooke Kalanick, explains the stubbornness of arm flab. She says in her book: 'Flab on the back of the arms can be indicative of low-testosterone levels. Females already have much lower testosterone levels than men, but many women can have even lower than normal levels due to stress or other common pitfalls, including:

- Inadequate protein intake
- Not lifting heavy enough weights
- Not training intensely enough (that is, doing long-distance, moderate-intensity cardio vs interval training with bursts/sprints)
- Lack of quality sleep
- Increasing estrogen exposure by eating hormone-laden meat and dairy, drinking out of plastic water

bottles, medications like birth control pills, and using cosmetics that contain parabens (common preservatives).'[1]

Who thought that stress and sleep could be related, right?

Also, upper arm fat can be caused by toxins in the body and also low testosterone levels, particularly in older women. But the most important cause is the simplest one—if you're overweight, you are more likely to have excess fat stores in your arms. Which only means that if you are overweight, you need to lose weight first, get down to what your body weight should ideally be and then start working on those arms. A holistic workout programme, that targets your entire body, is a must.

Thinking about wearing a sleeveless corset gown for the cocktail party? Or for your big bacherlorette? If yes, remember that your arms and neck will be up for display. For a bride or bridesmaid, toned arms are a great asset since most of the outfits at an Indian wedding show some amount of arm. The back parts of the arms are called triceps and these are the most affected areas on the arms. This is the region where fat is generally stored. All the exercises I've recommended can be done in the comfort of your home. So if you don't want a flash of flab at the wedding party, start with the exercises I've listed below. You'll have wonderfully firm arms in no time.

FAQ

Q: 'Nishi, if I work out my arms, will they get bulky?'

This is a common concern that most women have. They want toned arms sans the bulk. If you pump too much iron, then you will have Akshay Kumar-like arms, so use a moderate amount of iron in your workout and you should be fine and feminine!

A) Standing Exercises

1. The Butterfly

- Stand straight and raise your arms in front of you at shoulder level.
- Now raise your arms upwards and rotate it backwards and down and front again in a complete circle.
- Do this 20 times and then again 20 times backwards.

2. Chair Dips

- Find a stable chair, and stand with your back towards the seat.
- Take a step away from the chair, and bend your knees to the seat level.
- Bend your elbows and place them behind on the chair.
- Now dip down and touch your glutes to the floor. Your back should be straight the whole time.
- Repeat 20 or more times.

3. Beginning with Dumbbells

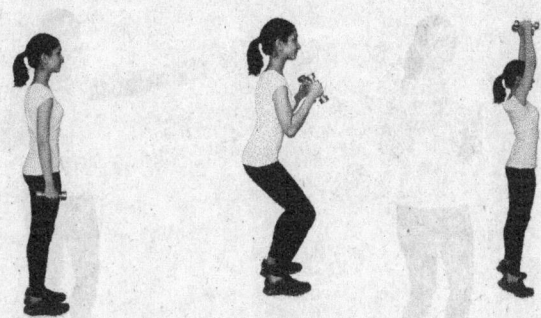

- Stand straight, holding a pair of dumbbells in your hands.
- Keep your body straight and lower it to the ground by bending your arms at the elbows.
- Now raise your body off the ground by extending your arms.
- Repeat 20 times.

4. Boxing with Dumbbells

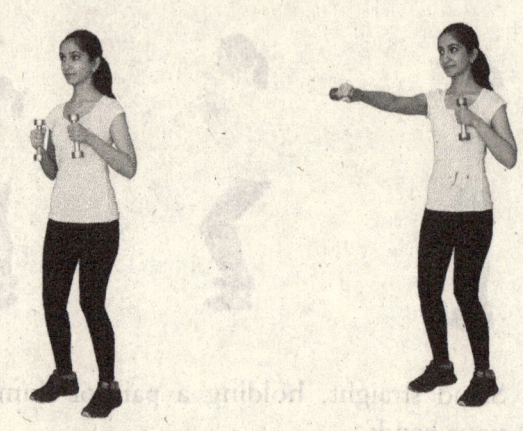

- Stand with feet slightly apart, and grab your dumbbells in each hand, palms facing each other.
- Punch your right fist up as high as possible without locking your elbow. Don't move your left fist.
- Pull the right fist back to the starting position as you punch your left fist upward.
- Do this for a minute. Remember to do this gradually. If it hurts, you must stop.

B) Floor Exercises

1. Table or Counter Push Ups

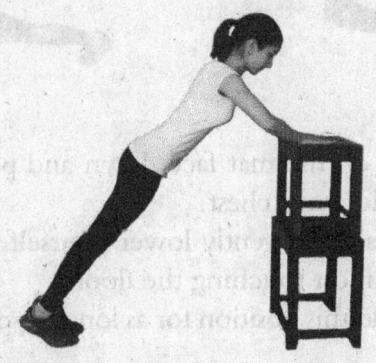

- Place your arms a shoulder-width apart on a table or kitchen counter that is stable.
- Gently push yourself down as if you were trying to hold a tennis ball between your shoulder blades. Your butt should be in a straight line and not sticking out.
- Hold this position for as long as you can and come up.
- Repeat 20 or more times.

2. Floor Push Ups

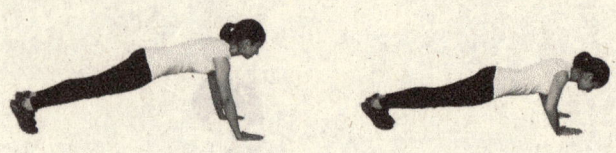

- Lie on the mat face down and place your hands under your chest.
- Inhale and gently lower yourself until your chest is almost touching the floor.
- Hold this position for as long as you can and come up.
- Exhale and bring your body back up to the starting position.
- Repeat 20 or more times.

3. Floor Dips

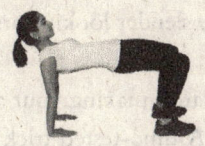 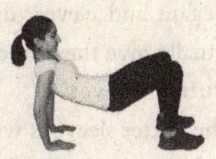

- Sit on the floor with your legs and feet pressed together, knees bent and feet firmly on the floor.
- Place your hands a little behind your butt, fingers pointing inwards towards your back. Straighten your arms to raise your butt off the floor.
- Bend your left elbow and lower your butt as close to the floor as possible without actually touching it.
- Straighten your left arm; repeat, this time bending your right arm.
- Alternate sides for 60 seconds.
- To make the move a little easier, try spreading your legs up to 2 feet apart.

Other activities

Skipping is another easy and convenient exercise that works wonders on your arms, because of the circular motion arm movement. In fact, skipping is one of the best cardio workouts there is. And it's cheap!

Sneaky Short-cuts

Have no fear, three quarter sleeves are here
Elegant and clever, dresses or shirts with three-quarter sleeves actually give the illusion of thinner, more slender looking arms.

Flutter sleeves
The flutter sleeve is wide and tapers upwards, making your arms look thin in their voluminous opening. A time-tested trick this one is.

Think long, think thin
Remember, the rule is that the shorter the sleeve, the more exposed your arm. So to cleverly hide these, opt for longer sleeves. If you don't want to be covered up, then try a dress with a lace sleeve. It's utterly classic and elegant.

Going sleeveless
And if you have a lovely new dress that's got spaghetti straps or is strapless, don't worry. You can hide away arm flab cleverly using scarves, wraps and shrugs that will immediately cover it up and that too, very stylishly.

Coming Up Next

The next chapter discusses the most common and persistent of all problem areas—the tummy. Workouts and cheat tricks will help you lose (and disguise) this area.

12

Belle and the Belly

'I have flabby thighs, but fortunately my stomach covers them'—**Joan Rivers**

The belly

Bane of both women and men.

And there's no love in love handles either.

I know for a fact that this particular area is the one that most brides-to-be fret about. And I can understand why. Whether you're wearing a sari or a lehenga, your tummy is the part of your body that's most highlighted. A flat, toned abdomen will look gorgeous and seamless in traditional Indian wedding wear. So if your tummy is a part that needs to be worked on, pay close attention to this chapter.

Abdominal fat is one of the most obstinate fat pockets in one's body. Not only that, it's unpleasant as hell to look at. Showing up as a tiny (or not) roll when

you sit, peaking out of tight-fitting T-shirts. But worst
of all is when you wear a sari. The sari highlights the
belly and waist and if you're not in shape then it isn't
the most flattering outfit. However, the sari is the most
worn outfit at weddings, and whether you are the bride
or not, you will most probably find yourself in one.
But please don't be disheartened. Even women who are
otherwise slender and fit and thin usually have a belly
that's visible due to underworked lower abdominal
muscles. I have to say this at the very outset—that it is
tough to remove abdominal fat especially, if the person
happens to be really obese. That being said, it is not
impossible. I've seen many clients over the past get
flat stomachs after working out regularly. With some
determination and patience, you too, could flaunt a flat
stomach.

Why do you get chubby around the tummy?
Some amount of belly fat is normal, it helps to cushion
the bones and organs and provide protection. Yet there
are three main reasons why you may accumulate fat in
the tummy region. These are:

1. **Metabolism**: According to a report by the Mayo
   Clinic, metabolism slows down as you age and this
   cause belly fat. Women are more prone to belly
   fat than men.[1] You must have noticed that some
   of your friends eat a lot of sugar-based foods, fried
   foods or cold drinks. Yet they manage to keep a
   flat stomach. The reason being, they have a very

high metabolism rate. If your metabolism is not good, you may have a bloated stomach. Thyroid conditions, diabetes and other medical conditions may perhaps be contributing reasons to slow metabolism.

2. **Sedentary lifestyle**: This point is fairly obvious. However, as simple as it sounds, it is 90 per cent of the reason. A sedentary life is a thriving platform for the accumulation of fat. So get off your couch immediately!

3. **Overeating**: Poor eating habits coupled with an excessive and sedentary lifestyle will obviously lead to a flourishing belly. According to medical experts, belly fat can be potentially dangerous. Excess of it can lead to a number of health problems including heart diseases, high blood pressure, Type 1 diabetes, a decrease in the level of HDL or good cholesterol, and can even lead to strokes or sleep apnea. You have to combat this problem before it gets too late.

Why belly fat is dangerous

According to the Mayo Clinic: The trouble with belly fat is that it's not limited to the extra layer of padding located just below the skin (subcutaneous fat). It also includes visceral fat—which lies deep inside your abdomen, surrounding your internal organs.

Although subcutaneous fat poses cosmetic concerns, visceral fat is linked with far more dangerous health problems, including:

- Cardiovascular disease
- Type 1 diabetes
- Colorectal cancer

Research also has associated belly fat with an increased risk of premature death—regardless of overall weight. In fact, some studies have found that even when women were considered a normal weight based on standard body mass index (BMI) measurements, a large waistline increased the risk of dying of cardiovascular disease.[2]

Correct posture

Before starting any exercise, remember to keep your posture straight.

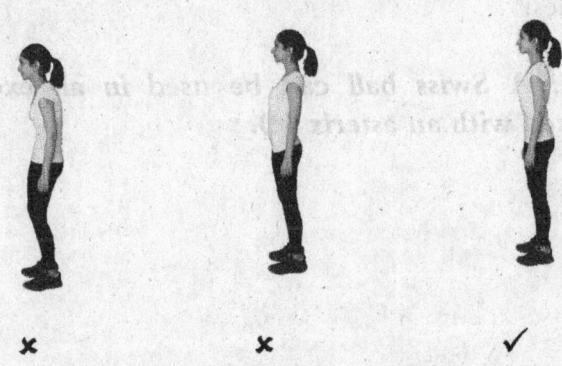

- Stand straight and firm with feet slightly apart.
- Keep your stomach pulled in with ease.
- Your chin should not be tucked into your neck. Make sure it's slightly pointed towards the ceiling. You should be able to hold a small ball between your neck and chin.
- Elbows should be tucked in, not out.
- Ensure that your breathing pattern is normal. While exhaling, push outwards with your abdomen and while inhaling, pull inwards with your abdomen.

This is a 20-minute workout of 10 exercises, divided into floor and standing exercises, that especially target belly fat and love handles. Do them regularly and you're bound to see those coveted abdomen muscles rise to the surface. Just remember to warm up and cool down after your workout. So what are you waiting for? Let's banish belly fat and say bye bye to those love handles!

Note: A Swiss ball can be used in all exercises marked with an asterix (*).

A) Floor Exercises

1. *Simple Crunch

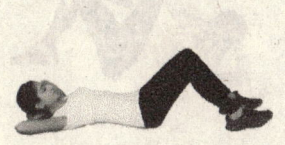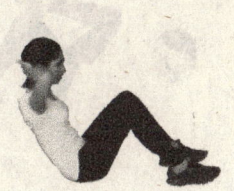

- Lie down flat on your mat with your knees bent and feet firmly planted on the ground. You can also lift your legs and place them on your Swill ball at a 90-degree angle.
- Lift your hands and place them behind your head or keep them crossed across your chest.
- Inhale deeply and as you lift your upper torso off the floor, exhale. As you lift your torso, do not sit up straight. You should be at a 30–40 degrees angle off the ground. Then only will you feel the pressure on your abdominal muscles.
- Inhale as you go back down and exhale as you come up.
- Do this at least 50 times. A 100 crunches is the ideal number per day.

2. Twist Crunch

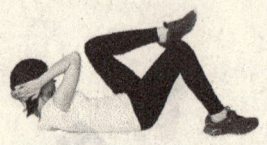 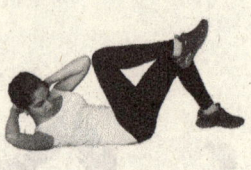

- Start from the supine position with your hands behind your head and your legs flat on the floor.
- Inhale deeply and lift your torso up, moving your right elbow towards your left knee. At the same time, bend your left knee and push it towards your right elbow. Try to touch them. If you can't that's okay. In time you will be able to do it.
- Exhale as you come back.
- Alternate with your left elbow.
- Do this at least 20 times.

3. Bicycle Crunch

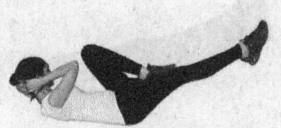 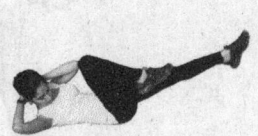

- Start from the simple crunch position.
- Now lift both your legs off the ground and bend them at the knees.
- Bring your right knee close to your chest, keeping your left leg out.
- Now take your right leg out and bring your left leg close to your chest.
- Alternate bending your knees this way as if you are paddling a bicycle
- Do this at least 50 times.

4. *Plank

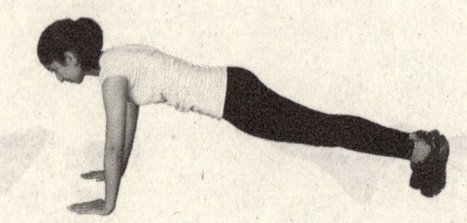

- Lie on your stomach with your hands placed by your chest.
- Push yourself up. Your hands should be directly under your shoulders, like you're about to do a push-up.
- Your toes and palms are the only parts that should be touching the floor. Remember, your glutes and back and head should be in a perfect incline. I should be able to roll a ball from your head to your toe without it falling off!
- Breathe normally. A lot of people forget to breathe when holding this position, a common mistake you should avoid.
- If you can, hold this position for 1 minute. With practice, you will be able to do it for a longer time.

You can also use your Swiss ball to do a plank by placing your hands on it.

- Draw your right knee towards your chest. Hold for one second, then return to the plank position. Repeat with your left knee.

5. Side Plank

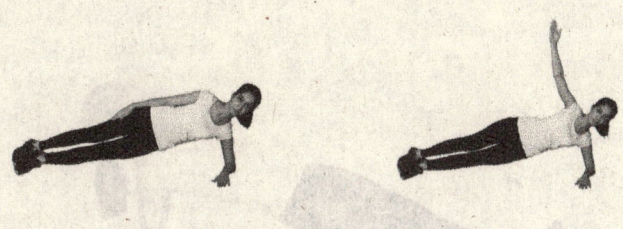

- Lie on your right side with your legs stacked one above the other.
- Inhale and push your body up, using your right arm strength.
- Stretch your left arm towards the sky.
- Keep your feet firmly on the ground.
- Look straight ahead and breathe normally.
- Again, keep in mind that your bum and abdomen should not stick out. They should be in a straight line.
- If you can, hold this position for 1 minute.

6. Reverse Plank

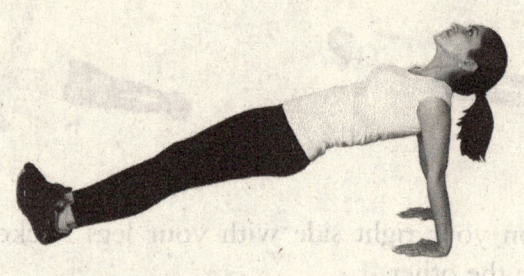

- Sit on your mat with your legs extended in front of you.
- Place your palms on the floor slightly behind your hips.
- Press down into the ground, pushing your hips up. Point your feet upwards, balancing on your heels.
- Squeeze your core and try to pull your belly button back towards your spine.
- If your hips sag or drop, lower yourself back to the floor.
- Look up at the ceiling but without straining your neck.
- If you can, hold this position for 1 minute.

7. Core workout

- Lie on your mat with your hands by your side.
- Exhale as you lift both your feet and arms a few inches off the ground.
- Focus your attention on your abs, forcing them to do most of the work to lift and lower your legs. Be sure to keep your lower back pressed to the floor the entire time.
- Hold this pose for as long as you can.

B) Standing Exercises

1. Side Stretches

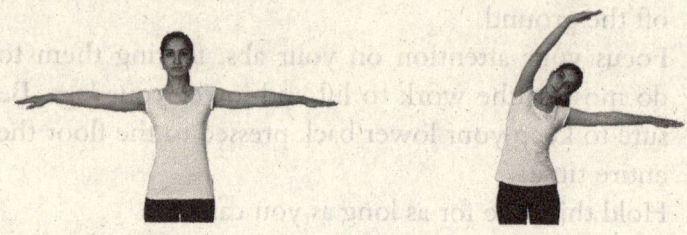

- Stand with your feet slightly apart.
- Stretch your arms out on both sides.
- Slowly bend to your right using your right arm to guide you. Do not put any pressure on it.
- Keep your left arm straight and aligned over your left ear. Look straight ahead.
- Hold this pose till you can and come up gently.
- Repeat on the other side.
- Do a set of 10.

2. Knee–cross Crunch

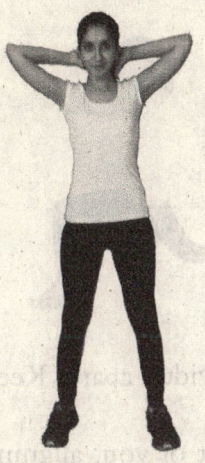
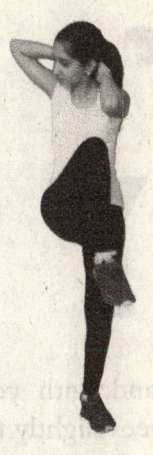

- Stand straight and extend your left arm up and your right leg to the side, toes pointed.
- Lower your left elbow and raise your right knee, crunching them together on a diagonal line. Return to the starting position.
- Do 15 on each side.

3. Lunges

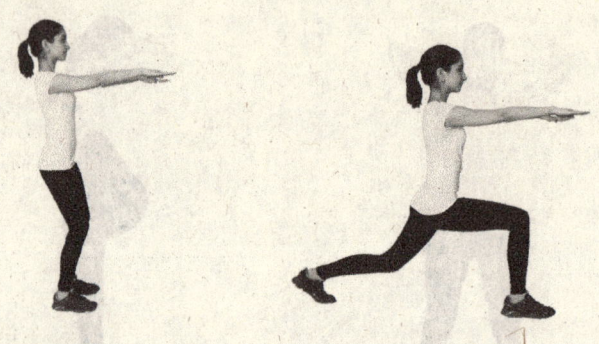

- Stand with your legs hip-width apart. Keep your knees slightly bent.
- Lift both your hands in front of you, aligning them with your shoulders and parallel to the ground.
- Take a big step forward with your right leg and sit down as if on a chair. The left leg should be positioned backwards supported by the toes.
- Keep your spine straight. Don't bend forward.
- Hold the pose and then bring your right foot back to its original place.
- Now do this with your left leg.
- Repeat 20 times.
- You can also use dumbbells while doing lunges. You will be working both your core and your arms if you do.

Sneaky Short-cuts

Do you want a flat stomach without any effort?

Invest in shapewear and a corset. Shapewear technology today can transform your body in seconds. From tummy tuckers to panties that can enhance your bottom to corsets that provide the perfect swell to your bosom, shapewear is every woman's modern-day saviour. Go for well-known brands, as their quality and results are always better than the cheaper stuff.

Think high-waist

A high-waist in both skirts and pants takes the eye away from the belly area.

Ditch the bodycon

Wear dresses that don't cling to you, which will reveal your tummy region. Instead, opt for structured, patterned or dresses with drapes.

Shift to shift

A shift dress is the perfect solution for those who want to hide a muffin top. It falls brilliantly and takes the eye away from one particular region. Asymmetrical dresses work well too, as they draw attention away from the belly and create a vertical line.

Horizontal stripes . . . be gone!

As a rule of thumb, never ever wear a dress with horizontal stripes. The optical illusion only increases your girth!

There's truth in layers

Layering your clothes helps to cover up unwanted sore sights and creates the illusion of a slim and lean figure.

The longer the better

A long top again creates the impression of a slimmer you. So go long over slacks and your jeans.

Coming Up Next

Next, we talk about your bottom and how you can firm it up with a workout routine.

13

The Bottom Line

'That thing there is something special'—**Puff Daddy** about
JLo's butt

Derriere me!

There is a universal dance little spoken about. It's the one women have invented and perfected over the years. The skinny-jean dance, I'd like to call it. Most of us do it as we're trying to wriggle into our favourite pair of jeans or a pair we covet at Zara. Oh! The wriggle and the struggle. And is going blue in the face and not eating when you have them on worth it when the zip is finally pulled up? Oddly, most women will say 'yes'.

After years of hate, the butt however, is making a comeback. An article in the *New York Times* says: 'The rear is fast becoming the erogenous zone of choice in America, vying for eminence with breasts, abs, legs or, for those of us who came of age in the early '90s, Linda Hamilton's sinewy arms in *Terminator 2*. Captivating back-end views of amply endowed personalities have stirred the popular imagination, prompting many women, it would seem, to chase after gawk-worthy curves of their own.'[1]

Then there's Jennifer Lopez, and the ostentatious rumours which claimed that she has had it insured for a whopping USD 27 million! She chose to celebrate her butt instead of losing it and in doing so provoked this lavish and rather colourful praise from *Vanity Fair* magazine who called her butt 'in and of themselves, a cultural icon'. Tina Fey writes in her book *Bossypants*: 'The first real change in women's body image came when JLo turned it butt-style,' she wrote. 'That was the first time that having a large-scale situation in the back was part of mainstream American Beauty. Girls wanted butts now. Men were free to admit that they had always enjoyed them.'[2]

But the truth is that the Botticelli Babe, once a dream figure, will take a lot of time to be accepted and desired in our size zero world. The bum is one of the trouble areas for most women. And particularly Indian women, as we are generally pear-shaped and tend to gain weight on the waist and hip below. If your lower body seems heavier than the rest of your body, it likely that that's where you store your excess fat. Genetics has a substantial role to play in it but mostly it is a sedentary lifestyle and wrong eating habits that allow fat to cling to this area. Some people have a higher number of fat cells present around the butt and thigh area. So if you are one of them, you need to take extra care to exercise correctly and shed the extra weight down there.

Know Your Bum

The muscles of the buttocks are known as the gluteals. The gluteals are composed of three muscle areas: the gluteus maximus, gluteus minimus and post glute medius.

Your glutes are the largest and perhaps most powerful muscle group in your body. And if you want to tone them, you need to first get off the couch, because sitting is not going to help!

Work your butt off

You need not be bummed out (pun intended) just yet because help is at hand. Every problem has a solution. I've set out eight exercises that target the bum region. But keep in mind that weight loss doesn't happen in just one region of your body. A workout programme should be aimed at the whole body. No single exercise or food will specifically burn fat from around your legs and bottom—your body does not discriminate when using fat for fuel. You must induce all-over weight loss. Once you start losing the kilos, you will notice a slimmer lower body. In the meantime, you can build muscle to create a more toned appearance in your problem areas. What these exercises *will* do, however, is tone and firm up a particular region.

There are many exercises to consider before beginning this mission. But I'm going to begin with squats. They are known as the 'king of all exercises' because squats are a complete workout routine in themselves, targeting the glutes, hamstrings, your core and quads. When done correctly, you can get a world of benefit from them— they will tone, firm and tighten your butt muscles, giving you a leaner lower body appearance. Because squats exercise all the biggest and major muscles of the human body they create more demand for energy production; thus energy expenditure is far greater when squatting than during any other exercise. In fact it's possible to burn a huge amount of energy within a very short time when maximum potential for the squat is reached. They also improve your coordination and balance. Plus, you can do them any time without the help of any equipment, although if you want to double the effect, you can add a dumbbell in the mix. So let's begin.

A) Standing Exercises

1. Squats

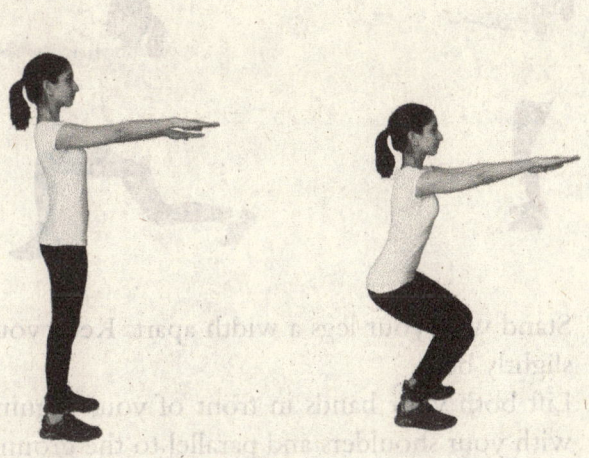

- Stand with feet your feet slightly wider than your shoulders.
- Extend your arms in front of you, palms facing down.
- Remember to keep your spine straight all the time.
- Inhale and bend your knees till you are in a squatting position.
- Look straight ahead and hold this position for a minute, if you can.
- Repeat 10 times.
- You could also hold a dumbbell to increase the effect. Beginners should avoid this.

2. Lunges

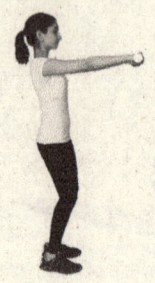 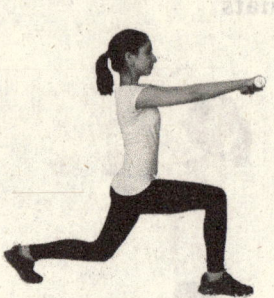

- Stand with your legs a width apart. Keep your knees slightly bent.
- Lift both your hands in front of you, aligning them with your shoulders and parallel to the ground.
- Take a big step forward with your right leg and sit down as if on a chair. The left leg should be positioned backwards supported by the toes.
- Keep your spine straight. Don't bend forward.
- Hold the pose and then bring your right foot back to its original place.
- Now do this with your left leg.
- Repeat 20 times.
- You can also use dumbbells, while doing lunges. You will be working both your core and your arms if you do.

3. Jumping Jacks

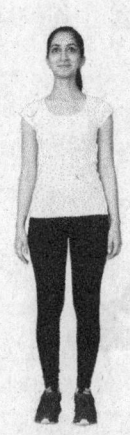 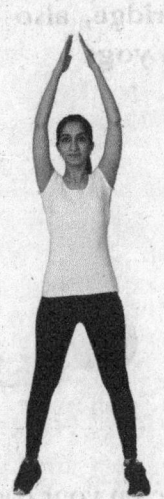

- Stand straight with your feet together.
- Jump, moving your feet shoulder width or slightly wider.
- At the same time, raise your arms up over your head with a clap. Your arms should be slightly bent throughout the entire in-air movement.
- Jump back to starting position.
- Try and do 100 of these if you can.

B) Floor Exercises

1. Bridge, also called Setu Bandha Sarvangasana in yoga

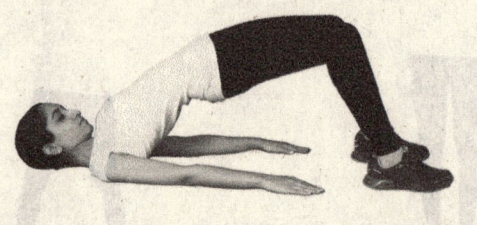

- Lie on your back on your mat with your arms flat on both sides.
- Bend your knees, keeping your feet firmly planted on the floor.
- Now gently raise your hips, arching your back as you do.
- As you come up, tighten your abdominal and buttock muscles.
- Hold this position for as long as you can.
- Gently come back to your starting position.
- Repeat 5 times.

2. Hip Raise—One Leg at a Time

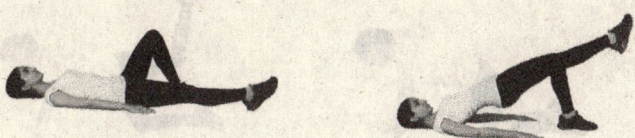

- Lie on your back on the mat with your left knee bent and your right leg straight.
- Raise your right leg until it is in line with your left thigh.
- Push your hips upward, keeping your right leg elevated.
- Hold this position for a while and then slowly lower your body and leg back to the start position.
- Do this 20 times, then repeat the same number of times with your right leg.

3. Glute Kickback

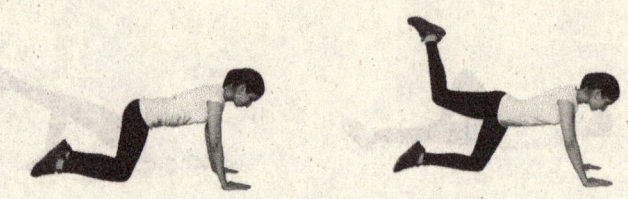

- Start with your hands and knees bent on the floor, spread out shoulder-width.
- Lift your right leg back and up. Your knee should be bent and your foot higher than your head.
- Squeeze your left glute and slowly lower your right back to your starting position.
- Do the same on your left leg.
- Repeat 20 times.

4. Exercise using your Swiss Ball

- Place yourself so that your abdomen is resting on the Swiss ball and your hands are on the floor on both sides. Your knees should be bent.
- Tighten your glute muscles and lift your right leg and hand off the floor, keeping them completely straight. Do not strain your back.
- Hold for a few minutes and come back to your starting position.
- Do the same on your left leg.
- Repeat 20 times.

5. Side Leg Raises

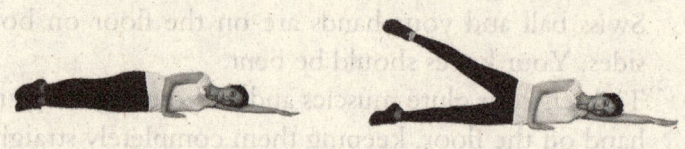

- Lie on your right side with your legs stacked one above the other and your left arm stretched out above your head. Your head should be resting on this hand.
- Now raise your left leg as high as you can, keeping your knees straight the whole time. Squeeze your glutes when you raise your leg.
- Hold for a few minutes and return to your starting position.
- Do the same on your right leg.
- Repeat 20 times.

Outdoor activities

To complement all your indoor exercises there are a few things you can do that will boost your overall workout programme and that works wonders for your bum. A few of these are as simple as climbing stairs, brisk walking, running and swimming. Try and add a few to spice up your routine. These are great ways to burn fat from your butt and body. For those of you who do not have a bicycle or live in a city where it's actually dangerous to ride a bike, just use the one at the gym.

Benefits of Brisk Walking

If hitting the gym is not your style, consider a brisk walk around your neighbourhood or park. A lot of people find walking a better alternative to gyms and a structured routine. It's more refreshing than an indoor workout programme, it helps clear the mind, it's the perfect beginner workout, and most importantly, it's free!

In fact, scientists at the University of Pittsburgh recently published a study where they found that overweight people who brisk walked for 30 to 60 minutes a day, lost weight without changing their other lifestyle habits.[3]

Walking fast will tone your glute muscles and thighs. Now give it a try!

Sneaky Short-cuts

Mean jeans
Opt for dark washes that immediately streamline your look.

Long tops
These tops have multi-value. They can hide a muffin top, like I said earlier, and at the same time their length beautifully hides away your derriere. A must have!

Palazzo pants
These wide-legged, flowing pants don't cling to your backside and create the illusion of length. Opt for a pair with smaller patterns though.

Bury it in cloth
A sari is the best fashion idea to hide away that backside. Layers and flowing length makes you look slimmer, creating the overall impression of a smaller behind.

Swear by shapewear
Once again, shapewear is the ultimate tool to bring shape and hold in your bum.

Fluff up that flat butt
Get pockets that are on an angle to give the illusion of shape; wear low-rise cuts to show off your waistline.
Don't: Go too baggy.

Coming Up Next

The next chapter will guide you through an exercise routine aimed specifically at your legs. Do the workout routine provided for slimmer and more toned pins.

The Bridal Diet

Coming Up Next!

The next chapter will guide you through my personal routine, which specifically for your legs. He the working routine provided for summarge and polished pins.

14

Shake a Leg

'The average man is more interested in a woman who is
interested in him than he is in a woman with beautiful legs'
—Marlene Dietrich

Two words: Sharon Stone.

I'm sure all of you remember the moment in the 1992 movie *Basic Instinct*, when Catherine Tramell (Sharon Stone) is being interrogated. It is a tense and gripping scene all right, but who can forget those legs? Conan O'Brien said on his show that: 'It is the most-paused moment'—in cinema history. Imagine what a pair of shapely and toned pins can do!

Long, shapely legs that stretch on forever are every woman's dream. They give you confidence and hold up your frame to perfection. However, not everyone is blessed with a pair that will go down in history. Most of us suffer from two common problems—thunder thighs and cellulite.

The reason behind thunder thighs is usually pinned on genetics but hormones can also play a part. Max

Tomlinson, author of *Target Your Fat Spots* and co-founder of MaxHealth explains thunder thighs, 'The female hormone oestrogen promotes fat storage around the top of the legs, and many of us are exposed to high levels of both natural oestrogens in water and farmed meat and synthetic versions—chemicals in plastics and non-stick coatings—in the environment.'[1]

What is Cellulite?

If you don't know the answer to that question, you're probably under twenty-five years of age or you work out every day like a horse or you're blessed with great genes. Because cellulite is very common. Even thin people have it. According to WebMD: 'Cellulite is nothing more than normal fat beneath the skin. The fat appears bumpy because it pushes against connective tissue, causing the skin above it to pucker.'[2]

We don't like this at all. Fat shouldn't 'pucker' or stand out or be seen! Worse still is that cellulite seems to appear without warning out of nowhere. *Prevention* magazine explains this brilliantly. 'You see less cellulite in men because their fibres run horizontally, forming a criss-cross pattern that prevents bulging or dimpling. Though cellulite can pop up any time, it is true that cellulite does seem to appear out of nowhere and get worse with age. That's because our tissues change. Those strands of connective tissue thicken with age, and our skin gets thinner, making cellulite more noticeable.'[3]

There's the long and short of it. With age, the problem worsens. So to fight off the fat you need to keep working out. Here's something very important that I wrote about at length in *Lose a Kilo a Week*. A lot of my clients ask me—If I exercise will my fat turn into muscle?

The answer is no. A lot of people confuse weight, muscle and fat.

Muscle and fat are two distinctly different tissues and one can't be turned into the other. Think of muscle as lead—heavy, dense and compact, whereas fat is as a sponge—voluminous and spreading. A person with more muscle could weigh more on the scales than a person with less muscle. Muscle will always be muscle and fat will always be fat. You can burn fat and build muscle. When you 'burn fat' you are actually shrinking the size of your fat cells by using the energy that has been stored there.

Understanding BMR

Now on to the other important part.

BMR or Basal Metabolic Rate is the rate at which your body burns calories when you're at rest. This is the minimum amount of calories that a body requires to stay alive. BMR can be responsible for burning up to 70 per cent of the total calories burnt.

Remember this: Your BMR decreases with age. After you turn 20, your BMR drops about 1 per cent every year. Every year, it becomes harder to eat whatever you want and stay slim. Every year, the job of staying fit and slim becomes 1 per cent harder. You've got to modify your eating accordingly as your body is slowing down. Your muscle build up is going down at the same rate and the bad news is that your fat mass goes up. So you should start eating 1 per cent less and exercise 1 per cent more every year.

However, all is not doom and gloom. With the right exercise routine, you can combat these unsightly fat pockets and keep them hidden where they belong. Here are a few exercises that target the legs. The truth is, many exercise routines simply don't include the key moves you need to truly target the often troublesome area of the inner thighs. Fortunately, slimmer, sexier, whistle-worthy legs can be yours in only a week or two if you follow these exercises sincerely.

1. Squats (see p 175 for reference)

- Stand with feet your feet slightly wider than your shoulders.
- Extend your arms in front of you, palms facing down.
- Remember to keep your spine straight all the time.
- Inhale and bend your knees till you are in a squatting position.
- Look straight ahead and hold this position for a minute, if you can.
- Repeat 10 times.
- You could also hold a dumbbell to increase the effect. Beginners should avoid this.

2. Squat Jumps

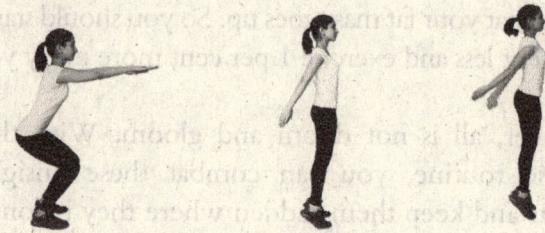

- Stand with your feet shoulder-width apart.
- Start by doing a regular squat, then engage your core and jump up explosively.
- When you land, lower your body back into the squat position to complete one rep. Land as quietly as possible, which requires control.
- Do 3 sets of 12 reps.

3. Sumo Squats

- Stand with your feet wider than hip-width apart, toes slightly turned out, holding a medicine ball in front of your chest.
- Squat down as low as you can, keeping your heels on the ground and your back straight.
- Press back up to standing. That's one rep.
- Do 3 sets of 12 reps.

4. Squat Kicks

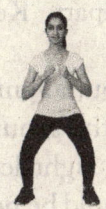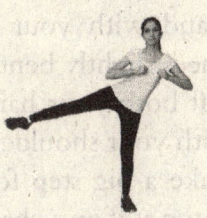

- Start in the squat position.
- Rise up, and kick your right leg straight out to the side at hip level.
- Return to the squat position and kick with the left leg.
- Do 15 on each side.

5. Lunges (see p 176 for picture)

- Stand with your legs hip-width apart. Keep your knees slightly bent.
- Lift both your hands in front of you, aligning them with your shoulders and parallel to the ground.
- Take a big step forward with your right leg and sit down as if on a chair. The left leg should be positioned backwards supported by the toes.
- Keep your spine straight. Don't bend forward.
- Hold the pose and then bring your right foot back to its original place.
- Now do this with your left leg.
- Repeat 20 times.
- You can also use dumbbells while doing lunges. You will be working both your core and your arms if you do.

6. Side Lunges

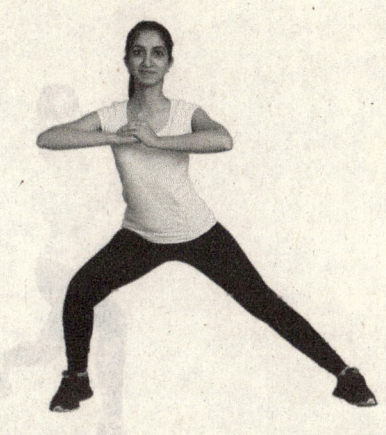

- Stand with your feet and knees together.
- Take a large step with your right foot to the right side and lunge towards the floor.
- Make sure your right knee does not extend past your toes and keep your left leg relatively straight.
- Push off through your right foot to return to the start to complete one.
- Do three sets of 12 on each side.

7. Skater Lunges

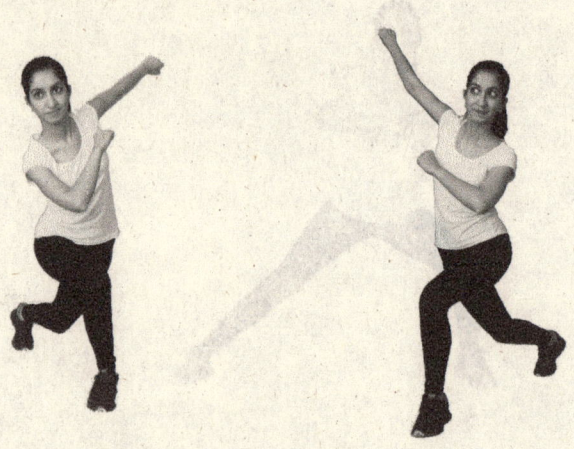

- From a standing position with feet shoulder-width apart, slowly step your left leg back diagonally behind your right leg.
- Lower into a lunge until your knee almost touches the floor.
- Return to standing and reverse the movement, stepping the right leg behind your left and lowering into the lunge.
- Complete 3 sets of 12 reps.

8. Standing Leg Curl

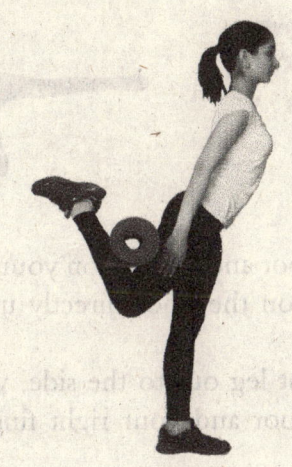

- Stand with your feet together and place a rolled-up mat evenly behind the right knee so that it's parallel to the floor.
- Lift your right foot behind you with toes pointed, and pull the heel towards your butt to secure the mat behind the knee.
- Extend your arms at shoulder level in front of you and clasp your hands. You can use a chair for balance.
- Squeezing the mat with your leg throughout, lean forward slightly, keeping your back flat, as you lift your right knee behind you a few inches lower.
- Do 20. Switch legs and repeat.

9. Side Kicks

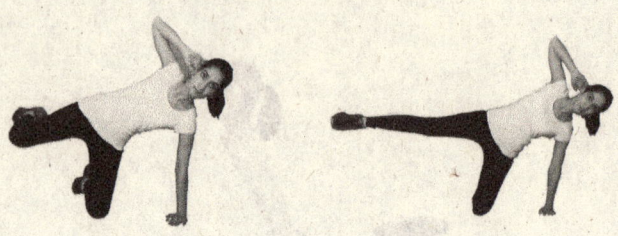

- Kneel on the floor and balance on your left knee with your left hand on the floor directly under your left shoulder.
- Bring your right leg out to the side, with your toes touching the floor and your right fingertips behind your head.
- Keeping your right leg straight, kick it forward at hip height, flex your right foot, then hold it for a second.
- Do 12 reps, switch sides, and repeat.

Sneaky Short-cuts

Going nude down there

By that I mean, getting yourself the perfect pair of nude shoes. Find a pair that matches your skin tone. Nude shoes give the impression of never-ending legs. They don't cut the feet off with a block of colour and create a slender physique. The same goes for nude nail polish!

Set the bar high

Wear anything with a high waist. Be it pants, jeans or skirts. A pair of high-waisted pants or shorts makes it seem as if your waistline's higher, and therefore, your legs longer.

Wide leg pants

Think 70s. Wide-leg pants, especially those with vertical details, are a smart way to elongate your size.

Get shorty

This one is simple enough. A short dress exposes more leg, making them look longer, especially if you're not that tall.

Swear by heels

Add heels to your footrobe. The extra few inches will give you the right swagger and make your muscles work too.

Empire state of mind

The empire line dress, especially the maxi, also creates a long and sleek illusion. You can maximize this by pairing it with a pair of wedges.

Coming Up Next

How many of us know women who have put on a ton of weight after getting hitched? I bet the answer is—all of us. Putting back the weight you've lost in the run up to your wedding is a very common problem worldwide. The next section helps you identify what factors lead up to post-wedding weight gain, and how you can be more aware and careful to keep extra weight at bay.

Part IV

Post-wedding

15

The Honey after the Moon

'[O]ur honeymoon will shine our life long: its beams will only
fade over your grave or mine'
—**Charlotte Brontë**, *Jane Eyre*

First of all I would like to say: Congratulations! You're a
married woman now and a whole new chapter of your
life is unfolding as you read these words. Or will you toss
this book aside, now that the wedding is over? I urge you
not to for many reasons. It's not to burst your bubble or
be a dampener in your happy time, but read on and you'll
find out why this is one of the most crucial chapters in
this book.

Here I look at some of the reasons why women gain
weight after marriage and it should help you to be aware
of what will come your way.

Bye Bye Single Life, Hello Weight—The Marriage Market Theory

Laila was on a strict diet up to her wedding. She had lost all the weight she wanted to and was looking hot and fit on the big day. She was the happiest bride if you saw her. Six months later, Laila comes to me and I barely recognized her. All the months of hard work had been unravelled. She had regained all her weight and more. 'What happened?' I asked her gently. To which she replied with a shrug, 'Marriage and in-laws.'

Gaining weight after the wedding is not uncommon. What happens after the stress and pressure of the wedding day is that diets become more relaxed and exercise takes a backseat now that the newlyweds no longer have a special event to be motivated by. A 2010 study that included more than 8,000 people over three years showed that fitness levels dropped in married people, while surprisingly, single women and divorced men got into better shape. Research says that this happens because of the 'marriage market' theory. Once people are married, they no longer feel the need to be perfect or in the best shape as they do not need to attract a mate. Since they already have one, they tend to slip back into old habits and routine. The motivation just flies out of the window.[1]

Playing Doubles

Marriage is the union of two people. It is also the coming together of two lifestyles—living habits such as sleeping, eating, hobbies, likes and dislikes. The time that was once only yours now becomes 'we time'. Women, especially, tend to prioritize their relationships over themselves and so it's not uncommon to see a woman skipping her morning run to spend time with her husband or giving him company when he watches TV. And there's nothing wrong with it, if she can find time to do the things she did before marriage. Cheryl Forberg, RD, nutritionist for *The Biggest Loser* and author of the cookbook *Flavor First* says, 'When you're combining lifestyles, sometimes the less active one wins out.'[2]

Eating for Two

Women are instinctive nurturers. They show their love and care to their family in many ways. And the most common way is to cook and feed them. Most newlywed women tend to go fancy while cooking. They want to both impress and delight their partner. Whether it's a simple but heavy pasta dish like spaghetti Bolognese or some Chinese, post-wedding cooking is almost always a lavish affair. Remember the days when you were single? What were your meals generally like? How easy was rustling up a sandwich? But a sandwich will not suffice when you're feeding a family. It's almost always a full spread. And naturally, the chances of gaining weight are tremendous.

The other factor is that men generally tend to eat much more because they need more calories than women for energy. *Fitness* magazine reports: 'The average active man needs up to 3,000 calories a day, compared with an active woman's 2,200, and his metabolism is 10 to 15 percent faster, which means he can put away bigger portions and not gain an ounce. The next thing you know, your plate looks like his does and your clothes are getting tight.'[3]

So it's very easy to fall into your husband's routine and lifestyle. And fall prey to the dangers of it by gaining a lot of weight.

Eating with Everyone

In India especially, there's the added factor of the in-laws and the extended family. Once you're married, you are invited to everyone's houses for introductions, which obviously centre around lunch or dinner—extravagant meals that are rich and high in calories. Refusing is tantamount to treason, so most brides (and grooms) tend to go the whole hog and indulge themselves. These are the days that matter the most. After watching your diet during the days leading up to your wedding, giving it all up will obviously make you put on weight. It's a slippery slope in healthy eating habits, which most women tend to fall prey to.

The Happiness Quotient

Dr Helen Fisher is a professor of love. As a biological anthropologist she is the author of five books about the evolution, expression and the chemistry of love, and has spoken at prestigious forums such as TED, World Economic Forum, South by Southwest. She says that, 'Romantic love, at its best, is a wonderful addiction. At its worst it leads to depression, suicide and even murder.

In fact, our brain scanning studies (using fMRI) show that when a person is in love, they exhibit activity in the same brain regions that become active when one is addicted to cocaine and other drugs, including the nucleus accumbens and the ventral tegmental area (VTA), two primitive parts of the brain involved in the production and distribution of dopamine. These infatuated lovers also show activity in the caudate nucleus, an ancient brain region that helps to integrate our thought and feelings. Dopamine is key. This neurotransmitter is the central component of the brain's reward system—the brain system that gives the lover focus, energy, motivation, and craving for the beloved. I can't think of any bigger reward than falling in love.

'Novelty drives up the dopamine system in the brain, and that gives you energy, which makes you more active and helps keep your weight down.'[4] And on the other hand, a serious and calm attachment like marriage increases oxytocin levels in the brain. Oxytocin is also called the 'love drug'. This is in place of dopamine and its rush. So what naturally happens is that you feel calmer, more at peace and unhurried about doing activities such as exercising.

What Then?
Now that you know the factors that drive up your weight post the wedding, you can be more aware of them. I'm not asking you to swat away relatives who invite you to lunch or ignore your husband. What you need to do is

to make sure you have your time—the time needed to care for yourself. It's the old rule that works best—'help yourself before you help others, fix your oxygen mask on before fixing others'. Because only if you're fit and healthy, can you be of any help to the people around you. Here are a few points to incorporate and be mindful of in the days to come:

1. **Scheduling your day**: As much as you want to skip your daily exercise, I urge you not to. Maintaining your daily quota of cardio (even if it's just 20 minutes) will go a long way. Don't feel guilty for going out on your run. It's absolutely okay to do so. You'll have a more successful relationship if you're happy and fit. Remember, fitness boosts your confidence, self-esteem and your sex life. So now do you really want to miss your 20 minutes?

2. **Plan activities together**: If you're not keen on continuing with your workout routine, find activities that you can do together. Ask him what he's interested in and tell him what you like. You could be surprised by the answers. If he likes rock climbing and you like salsa—make a compromise. Set out days for both activities. This way you'll also increase your bond with each other.

3. **Lead by example**: If your husband isn't too keen on getting off the couch, lead by example. Only you can motivate him off that couch and show him

how much fun physical activities can be. After all, you don't want both of you sinking into a heavy and sluggish life, do you? Once he sees how active and fit you are, I can guarantee he'll be following you. Like I keep saying, it's only results that motivate a person. Show them that, and you're halfway there.

4. **Portion control**: Your husband's plate is always going to be bigger than yours. That's because he needs more energy than you. Keep this in mind every time your plate starts looking like his. If necessary, get yourself a smaller plate so that it naturally restricts the amount of food you pile on it. You don't need to starve yourself. Being healthy is about a balanced and nutritious diet, so as long as you have all the goodness of life (and that doesn't mean chocolates) on your plate, you can do perfectly well with a smaller one.

5. **Restricting TV time**: TV is a huge culprit in weight gain. Most newlyweds tend to bum around and watch endless TV, things they perhaps didn't bother to watch when they were single. Because TV time is generally considered 'together' time. Suggest other ways to bond instead of hours of mindless TV. It could be anything like going to an art gallery, going shopping, taking classes together.

In closing, I would like to wish you the best—the best marriage, the best family, the best years of your life. I wish you all of these and more. But none of this is truly possible without the best health. A healthy and happy person can achieve much more than someone who isn't. Keep this in mind always. Treat your body like the temple it is, and watch the rewards pile up on your plate. And if you slip, after all you're only human, don't be afraid to kick back up and start again. Life is about going forward and falling back. It's the way things work. If we didn't fall we would never learn from them. Trust me, I've battled Type 1 diabetes all my life, and I've fallen and risen higher. There's nothing we can't do with our bodies. We take it for granted most of the time, but one day the signs of damage will show. So don't wait till that happens. Take control, seize back the power that is yours. Human beings are a resourceful lot; that's why we're on top of the food chain, an evolutionary miracle. We've conquered the world and the skies. So what's a little healthy living compared to all of that? The answer is: nothing. It's the simplest changes we make in our life that will serve us in the years to come.

So here's to a healthy, happy and blessed marriage. To you, my beautiful readers.

References

Chapter 1
Heavier Ever After and Other Troubles

1. Quoted from an article titled 'City of 100,000 Weddings', http://www.rediff.com/getahead/slide-show/slide-show-1-specials-city-of-100000-weddings-delhi-gears-up-for-the-shaadi-season/20111125.htm.
2. Quoted from an article titled 'Band, Bajaa, Bride', http://businesstoday.intoday.in/story/indian-wedding-business/1/21744.html.

Chapter 3
The Beautiful Bride Programme

1. McNaught, Judith, *A Kingdom of Dreams,* Simon and Schuster, May 1991.
2. Quoted from an article titled 'How Sleep Loss Adds to Weight Gain', http://well.blogs.nytimes.com/2013/08/06/how-sleep-loss-adds-to-weight-gain/?_r=1.
3. Gaardner, Jostein, *Sophie's World,* Farrar, Straus and Giroux; Reprint edition, March, 2007.

References

4. Quoted from an article titled '14 Ways to Cut Portions Without Feeling Hungry', http://www.health.com/health/gallery/0,,20769037,00.html.
5. Quoted from an article titled 'Want To Curb Your Appetite And Stop Sugar Cravings? Then Put These On Your Grocery List', https://beautifulbeginnings.wordpress.com/eating-healthybalances-your-diet/.
6. Quoted from an article titled '15 Foods to Help You Lose Weight', http://www.chron.com/life/healthzone/slideshow/15-foods-to-help-you-lose-weight-73562/photo-5426413.php.
7. Quoted from an article titled '8 Secret-Weapon Foods for Weight Loss You Should Eat this Year', http://read.plash.in/2015/01/01/8-secret-weapon-foods-weight-loss-eat-year/.

Chapter 4
I Do . . . Not
1. Gray, Claudia, *Evernight*, HarperTeen; 1 Reprint edition, October 2009.
2. Quoted from an article titled 'Positive Reinforcement', http://www.educateautism.com/behavioural-principles/positive-reinforcement.html.

Chapter 9
Up in Arms
1. Quoted from an article titled 'How Do I Get Rid of Arm Flab?' http://www.shape.com/celebrities/star-trainers/ask-celeb-trainer-how-do-i-get-rid-arm-flab.

210

Chapter 10
Belle and the Belly

1. Quoted from an article titled '17 Simple Exercises to Reduce Belly Fat', http://www.stylecraze.com/articles/5-exercises-and-5-foods-to-reduce-belly-fat/.
2. Quoted from an article titled 'The Belly Fat: What Your Waistline May Say About Your Health', http://www.mayoclinic.org/documents/healthsource-pdf/doc-20079413.

Chapter 11
The Bottom Line

1. Quoted from an article titled 'For Posterior's Sake', http://www.nytimes.com/2014/09/18/fashion/more-women-seeking-curvaceous-posteriors.html?_r=0.
2. Fey, Tina, *Bossypants*, Reagan Arthur / Little, Brown; Reprint edition (29 January 2013).
3. Quoted from an article titled 'Forget the Gym: Why a Brisk Walk is Really the Best Workout', http://batroypol.blogspot.in/2012_10_01_archive.html#.VSUAeNyUfNw.

Chapter 12
Shake a Leg

1. Quoted from an article titled 'Where Is Your Battle of the Bulge?', https://www.questia.com/newspaper/1G1-372064923/where-is-your-battle-of-the-bulge-bingo-wings-love.
2. Quoted from an article titled 'Cellulite', http://www.webmd.com/beauty/cellulite/cellulite-causes-and-treatments.

3. Quoted from an article titled '6 Moves That Target Stubborn Cellulite', http://www.prevention.com/fitness/strength-training/6-moves-target-cellulite.

Chapter 13
The Honey after the Moon
1. Quoted from an article titled 'Happily Ever Fatter? How to Avoid Post Wedding Weight Gain', http://www.fitnessmagazine.com/weight-loss/tips/avoid-weight-gain-after-marriage/.
2. Quoted from an article titled 'Legally Muscled', http://legallymuscled.blogspot.in/2013/11/marriage-and-weight-gain.html.
3. Ibid. 1.
4. Quoted from an article titled 'Anthropologist and Love Expert Helen Fisher on the Mysteries of Love', http://www.elsevier.com/connect/anthropologist-and-love-expert-helen-fisher-on-the-mysteries-of-love.

Acknowledgements

I was inspired to write this book after dealing with many of my clients who came to me with a dream of looking beautiful and svelte on their 'big' day. Invariably, most of them were dealing with a lot of pressure to look their best in a relatively short period of time. This book draws on the collective experience of helping these brides-to-be. I would like to acknowledge these clients and thank them for the trust and faith that they placed in me.

I would like to thank my parents who have given me their unconditional support and have allowed me to be the person I am today. Over the past years, with the progressive nature of juvenile diabetes, I have faced many challenges and some very difficult times when I was unable to perform even my day-to-day functions. Thanks to the support of my family, and especially my parents, I have been able to deal with my medical and other challenges in life and lead a relatively normal life. I am greatly appreciative of my father's medical advice and insight, which has enabled me to experiment and come up with different ideas around health and fitness.

Acknowledgements

My mother's persistent and unconditional support and guidance has enabled me to tirelessly pursue my work. I am extremely grateful to them for dedicating their lives to me. Without them, my work and this book would not be possible.

Other people that I would like to acknowledge and thank are my sister Neelima and her daughter Saachi, my brother Barun and sister-in-law Anita, my cousins Neetoo, Ritu, Madhu, Salil, Dr Gautam Kumar, my mentor Dr Kamlesh Vasudeva, and all my staff, including Usha, Nisha, Annu, Kiran and Sheela. Without their love, support and guidance, I wouldn't have been able to write this book.

Finally, a big thank you to all my clients for believing in me and for giving me another opportunity with this book. I love you all.

A Note on the Author

Nishi Grover is a dietician, who has had over 1500 clients until now at her clinic in south Delhi. She started her career as an aerobics trainer in 1988, and today charts out personalized diet plans (a combination of diet, exercise, and weight loss therapies) for her clients. She also has a low-cal café where her clients can gorge on goodies like apple tarts, kulfi, shahi tudkas and chocolate cakes—made without sugar or oil.

She is the author of the bestselling book *Lose a Kilo a Week*.